Slow Burn

Burn Fat Faster
By Exercising Slower

Stu Mittleman
with Katherine Callan

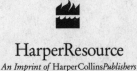

HarperResource
An Imprint of HarperCollins*Publishers*

To Fred Lebow, whose passion for running was only exceeded by the love he generated in the lives of those he touched.

HarperCollins books may be purchased for educational, business, or sales promotional use. For information, please write to: Special Markets Department, HarperCollins Publishers Inc., 10 East 53rd Street, New York, New York 10022.

First HarperResource paperback edition published 2001.

Designed by William Ruoto
Illustrations by Rick Johnson

Library of Congress Cataloging-in-Publication Data

Mittleman, Stu, 1951–
    Slow burn : burn fat faster by exercising slower / Stu Mittleman
and Katherine Callan.
      p. cm.
    Includes bibliographical references and index.
    ISBN 0-06-273674-4 (pbk.)
    1. Self-actualization (Psychology) 2. Running. 3. Marathon running. I. Callan,
Katherine. II. Title.
BF637.S4 M58 2000
613.7—dc21   99-048467

05 ❖/RRD 10 9 8 7

Contents

Contents

Before You Set Out . . .

The rest of your life begins today—and what a great day it can be! The power you need to create anything you desire already lies within you. All you need to do is tap into your body's innate wisdom to generate the energy that will carry you through. The process is neither mysterious nor complicated. It has to do with how you think, train, and eat. Once you master it, you will travel along the road ahead, calmly, confidently, and with eager anticipation. No matter what happens, you will remain positive, strong, and able to handle whatever comes your way. Enjoy the process of learning. Use the experience of physical training to get in touch with your body and learn as much as you can about yourself.

As you prepare to begin, let me remind you of what may sound like plain old common sense. No one should begin an exercise program without first obtaining medical clearance, especially if you have a personal or family history of heart disease, high blood pressure, or if you are over age 40, have diabetes, high cholesterol, smoke cigarettes, are overweight, or are taking medication. If you notice signs of overexertion or heart problems, such as pain or pressure in the left or mid-chest area or left neck, shoulder, or arm, lightheadedness, cold sweat, unusual paleness or fainting, stop exercising and seek medical attention. Overexertion can cause serious injury, including heart attack. Some individuals cannot safely elevate their heart rate to the levels typically used in heart-rate training zones. If you are unsure about your current health status or have any questions, contact your health care provider before you begin.

Armed with the necessary clearance, you're free to focus on the process of movement and move another step closer to mastering your physical destiny.

Acknowledgments

This book represents the culmination of a journey that began when I first ran up Flagstaff Mountain in Boulder, Colorado, on New Year's Day in 1977. Little did I know then where the road I was on would take me, but it sure was a lot farther than I could have ever imagined. What I thought would be a brief interlude in my life became my life. Now, more than twenty years later, I'd like to recognize the people who have contributed their support along the way.

I thank my mom, Selma, and dad, Irv, who always encouraged me to seek my own way and follow my convictions, even if others didn't always understand what I was trying to do—I only hope I can be as selflessly loving and supportive of my children as they are with me; my sister Jan, I offer thanks for her unwavering belief in me, especially during those times when I began to doubt myself; my uncle Herbie, who was the first great athlete I ever met; my teachers and advisors, Marlin Mackenzie, Bernard Gutin, and Ronald DeMeersman of Columbia University and Warren Ramshaw, Coleman Brown, and Doc Berry of Colgate— I am grateful for all the wisdom you have shared with me, the values you instilled in me, and the high standards to which you held me; my coaches, running buddies, and friends; my first running coach, Norman Fink, who also was my high school English teacher, for the funny hats you made us wear and the songs you let us sing as our cross-country "gang" went out for our longer train-ing runs and for teaching me to remember to smile and enjoy myself as I run; Brian Flanagan, who for years supported me at races, never let me get down, and always knew how to keep me moving forward; Brian Jones, for suggesting that I run my first ultra two weeks after the 1978 New York City Marathon; Leslie Holland, for persuading and encouraging me to start this project in the first place; my good friends Murry Zborowski, Glen Ezekiel, and Ray and Donna Charron, for reveling with me in the good times and sticking by me when times weren't so good; all my clients, for being inspirational and extraordinary. This has been both a joyous and arduous process—a different kind of thousand-mile race. I am confident that because of it, I can be an even more effective coach and teacher and we will all stand to benefit.

I want to especially acknowledge Anthony Robbins, who inspired me to keep raising the bar and reach for the stars. Tony, it was you who convinced me that what I had to say mattered and that I had more to offer than just a strategy to keep putting one foot in front of the other. I also want to thank his wife, Becky, who reminded me that sometimes movement and exercise can simply mean a moment to be alone with yourself and indulging in the pleasure of your own thoughts. Not everything has to be couched in terms of its impact on productivity and performance. Sometimes feeling good is enough of a reason.

I thank Gavin de Becker and Gary Shandling for the time you spent listening to me ramble on about my early ideas for this book and for the invaluable suggestions you offered to help me move my book along. I also am grateful to my editor, Robert Wilson at HarperCollins, and my agent, Simon Green, for having the vision to make this book possible.

Phil Maffetone, a kind and gentle soul, gave my running career new life, my intellect new perspective, and my life new meaning. You have forever changed the way I think about health and fit-ness. I benefited from the humble brilliance of Dr. Robert Young and his wife, Shelly. My wife, Mary Beth, and I are so happy we have had the great fortune to have met you and realize we all share in a mission to spread the "inner light" about health. Thank you Pete and Troi Egoscue, who listened to my vision for this book and immediately knew that I was communicating a message for living a life without limits.

John Maguire, Herbie Ross, Dr. Tom Crais, Nate Zinsser, and Sam Georges—you have all been dear friends and mentors. I cherish your involvement in my life on so many levels. You have been generous with your time, understanding, and patience. Thank you for being my friends.

The ideas of Peter D'Adamo, whom I have never met, have had such tremendous impact on my work. His contributions to the world of health and fitness are powerful. I am grateful as well to Dina Khader, who studied with D'Adamo and so graciously donated her time to educate my client base and me on the power of the blood-type distinction in food choice.

To my cowriter, Katherine Callan, I can only say, you are amazing. To have worked with me through all the late nights, the long hours, and the coast-to-coast phone conversations is remarkable. Your buoyant spirit, uncontrollable passion for the project, and commitment to do whatever it took to complete this was infectious. It was a complete joy to work with you.

To my beautiful and brave wife, Mary Beth, I thank you for supporting me with strength, courage, and determination and challenging me to stick with this process to the very end. There were times when I felt on the verge of not seeing this through, and you were there to help me stay the course. Your relentless and unshakable sense of optimism and hope is a gift. I am truly blessed. Finally, to my children Beau and Mackenzie. My heart and soul belong to you. You are the energy in my heart, and the light that continues to illuminate the road ahead.

*"There is no passion to be found playing small—in settling for a life
that is less than what you are capable of living."*

—Nelson Mandela

I remember when I first heard about a man who had run a
thousand miles in just over eleven days. My initial thought was,
"What a lunatic!"

My second thought was, "I have to meet this guy. I need to
understand the distinctions he has made that have allowed him
to achieve this unbelievable breakthrough. How was he able to
do it? How did he average three marathons a day for nearly
twelve days? How was it possible for him to feel stronger at the
end of the run than at the beginning? Perhaps most importantly,
what could I learn from what he had done?"

Over the past ten years Stu Mittleman has given me an educa-
tion in physical mastery. The initial outcome I was trying to
reach was fairly simple: I wanted to take the stress out of exercise.
For years I had severe back pain, which made running nearly
impossible. I was missing the joy of moving with grace and
power.

In a broader sense I wanted to maximize my body's potential. I wanted to be in a peak physical state. I wanted to be strong, I wanted to be lean, and I wanted to have endless energy. With Stu's guidance, I achieved the outcomes of a peak physical state and endless energy and enjoyed the process.

One of my core beliefs is that if you want to experience success in a given field, you must study the leaders in that field. Not only must you study these experts, you must learn what separates them from others. You must model their actions to achieve a similar degree of success. Stu Mittleman is the person I want to model in physical health.

Let me ask you this: If you wanted to learn about investing, would you study your next-door neighbor who dabbles in the stock market over the Internet? Or would you want to learn from Peter Lynch or maybe Warren Buffett? You probably would want to learn from the best of the best and implement their techniques, strategies, and philosophies.

Slow Burn is your chance to model Stu Mittleman. By picking up this book, you have the opportunity to learn from someone who not only has two postgraduate degrees and has conducted doctoral work in applied physiology, but who also has applied his knowledge base to make himself the preeminent ultraendurance athlete of our time.

Maybe your goal is not to be a world-class ultraendurance athlete but to prepare for the marathon of life. Your foundation is your physical state. Your physiology—your physical body—radically affects your mental state. Everything that we feel is a result of the way we use our bodies. The way we move affects the way we think, feel, and behave. Movement—everything from running, clapping, or jumping to the smallest movements in the muscles of the face—affects our body's chemistry. To put it another way, emotion is created by motion.

Slow Burn will teach you how to move aerobically, burn fat, and eat foods that support a healthier lifestyle. Ultimately, *Slow*

Burn will teach you how to prepare your body—and your mind—to go the distance in life.

Live with passion!

Anthony J. Robbins

Author of *Unlimited Power* and *Awaken the Giant Within*

Introduction

Physical training is more than just a means to an end; it can be an end in itself. For me, the movement is the reward. Many people I work with have a specific outcome in mind when they start a training program. Some want to lose weight, build muscle, or get rid of excess body fat. Others want to improve sports or personal performance. Most start out excited about realizing their goals so they can feel great about themselves later. The point Slow Burn makes—indeed the primary question it asks—is why wait?

This book is a journey of self-discovery through movement, especially running and walking. It's about learning to make decisions that empower you in the moment you make them. It's about generating choices that bring you joy and pleasure the moment you make them. It's about having every day and every moment filled with self-discovery, self-awareness, and self-fulfillment.

This book is not a step-by-step plan, written by someone else for someone else. It's about using running to become so integrated with your body, so aware of what it is your body wants and needs that you become confident in every decision—how much, how often, and how intensely you must move and what you eat, in what combination, amount, and frequency—that you become the master of your own physical destiny. The promise is that you will be self-guided and learn to make great decisions based on what's best for you.

You can have what you want *now*. You don't have to focus on a point in the future, and you don't have to work to get anywhere other than where you are. Because it is only when you're able to live in the moment and be guided by the clues your body is giving you that you can go out and accomplish everything you've ever imagined—and more.

I'm at Anthony Robbins' Date with Destiny seminar in Florida when I meet a talented marathon runner named Brittany. She's qualified for the prestigious Boston Marathon at 3 hours and 15 minutes. She suggests we go for a run. At first, I am hesitant. Since completing my journey across America in Spring 2000, I have been running 12-minute miles—nowhere near the seven-minute-per-mile-pace Brittany is accustomed to. But as the seminar is coming to a close, I decide her request is a good idea—"for one hour, and at an easy, comfortable pace." She agrees, and we make plans to meet the following day.

The morning is incredible—the sun is shining, and walkers, runners, and strollers are moving up and down a boardwalk that runs along the clean sand beach and magnificent deep blue ocean.

"Would you mind if we start off walking?" I ask. She agrees. We begin walking and talking. Brittany asks me "at what pace do I usually train?" This sets me off on a rather long soliloquy about what it is I focus on when I run.

"The point for me is not to focus on the pace I am running, but on the experience I am having," I share. "The important thing for me is how effectively I manage my 'state,' not how fast I run." I explain that what is really important to me is that my body is burning fat—not sugar—as an energy source. I constantly monitor my experience as I move: What do I see? What is it I hear? How do I feel? I then "chunk down" these distinctions even further, relaying the fundamental distinctions that make up the heart and soul of my *Slow Burn* perspective.

"Each energy-producing state has specific and real sensory-based references. When you move you are burning mostly fat, mostly sugar, or you are somewhere in between. Your body knows this by the way the world 'looks,' 'sounds,' and 'feels.' When you move in a comfortable fat-burning state, the visual information is distinct, expansive, and three-dimensional with a peripheral vastness and expansiveness that is unique and identifiable. It's as though you are in a 3-D surround-vision movie theatre." I describe the scene unfolding before us as we move from an easy walk to a jog and finally into a comfortable run.

"On the other hand," I continue, "as you shift into a more challenging sugar-burning state, visual information tends to collapse inward, the peripheral fringes tend to disappear and your attention gets drawn into a much narrower field of vision. Visual images flatten out, become two-dimensional, and you begin to feel as though you are running through a tunnel with the world painted on the inside walls. The same is true of the sounds and feelings you have as you move. Each set of sensory-based information changes depending on the energy-producing state in which you are moving. I constantly monitor my experience, increase my awareness, and base my decision on whether to 'speed up' or 'slow down' on these visual, auditory, and kinesthetic references."

Brittany had never heard running described in this way. She nearly comes to a complete halt to process and integrate what she has just heard. "You know, Stu, for me, running has always been about how fast I could go," she says. "I get my running gear on, lace up my shoes, and place 'blinders' over my eyes and 'just do it!' I am not at all present to the sights, sounds, and feelings you described. My head is down, my focus is on getting the job done. My experience is one of effort and strain while I am running and relief when it is over. Now that I have experienced running in this way I realize how much enjoyment—even spiritually—I have been missing. I thank you, for I know that my experience of running will now never be the same."

As she is speaking, Brittany's physiology changes dramatically. She is more relaxed, she is smiling from ear to ear, and her eyes glow like radiant jewels. She is happy, and tells me how great she feels right in the moment. She realizes how caught up she was in not letting herself feel good until her goals were met. Even then, she was so used to focusing on her goals that even when she achieved them the joy and happiness, excitement and contentment lasted only moments. She was used to living in the past or future; in the present she did not have a strategy for choosing to feel great.

The condition of your body—and ultimately the feelings of energy, vitality, excitement and joy you can expect to experience on a day-to-day basis—is solely determined by the kinds of decisions you make about what you eat, how you train, and what you focus on. You will never make the best decisions for you and your body on a consistent basis if you don't know what to "look," "listen," and "feel" for. This book, *Slow Burn*, can provide this for you. It is my gift to you, the product of over twenty years of research and personal experience.

Life is a marathon, not a sprint, and you must prepare accordingly. Unlike sprinters, who focus on how fast they can get to the finish no matter the cost, endurance athletes have no finish line. There is only the present moment, in which they must remain connected to their body, in tune with their every move, in a place that feels comfortable and productive and that they are able to maintain indefinitely.

People today have challenges that are comparable to an endurance event that seemingly never ends. We have to get up earlier, work longer hours, and attempt to carve out high-quality family or personal time over the course of the ever-increasing chaos of a day. Then we have to wake up the next day and do it again; and again and again and again . . .

To be productive in the long run of life, you have to pace yourself in order to feel strong, alert, and energetic. With the right pace, mindset, and diet, anything is possible: constant energy, feeling as strong at the end of the day as when you started out, and maintaining a consistently positive attitude.

For most of my life, I've been a professional endurance athlete, and now, like you, I am participating in the marathon of life. I still run every day, manage a business, and raise a family with my wife, Mary Beth. Running gives me the energy to do this. No matter what's going on in my life, I run a couple of hours a day, not because I think I have to or feel that I must, but because I am certain that when I am moving, I will feel great. I also know that after I run, I will have even more energy for the rest of my day. I'll be able to think more clearly, concentrate better, and feel more relaxed and at ease. When I'm in this state, anything—and everything—is possible. The experience is magical. I consider it a gift, one that ignites my life's mission, which is to get people to transform movement from "another task to complete" into an act that is so absolutely satisfying they can't imagine not having it as a regular part of their lives.

I recognize that in order to receive the gift that running offers me, I have to commit some of my time. Yet in this instance, the relinquishing of time actually creates more time. An hour set aside for generating reliable and everlasting energy frees up two to three or more hours in a day that might have otherwise been allocated to rest, recovery, or sleep. Suppose you could sleep less yet feel even more rested and alive—what would you do with the extra hours that suddenly appeared in your day? What if you could make your rest and recovery cycles more effective and get rid of those periods during the day when your energy wavers and your ability to concentrate wanes? How much more productive might you be if instead of daily lulls you experienced a steady stream of calm and enduring energy, mental clarity, and physical well-being? What if your day-to-day life became a cornucopia of energy and time? In this brave new world of endurance living, energy creates time, communication with your body leads to action, and the sheer pleasure of moving provides the motivation.

My career takes me all over the world and affords me the opportunity to coach thousands of people, from grandmothers to CEOs. Some people come to me because of my success in the world of endurance sports, others because of my affiliation with the extraordinary Anthony Robbins. I remember vividly when Tony first brought me to his Life Mastery seminar in March of 1992. He seemed less amazed by my world record for running a thousand miles than by the fact that I looked and felt better at the finish than before I started. Because of this, he thought that I could contribute something special about what it takes to go the distance and feel great doing it to the thousands of participants at his seminars. He gave me the opportunity to share with his clients the same lessons I am about to share with you.

I believe you can always take another step and do a little more, naturally and without stress. How can you accomplish this? Your body already knows. All you need to do is to become tuned in to the messages it has always been sending you about what it wants and how it can most benefit. Listen to your body and follow its wisdom. Marvel at the satisfaction you get from knowing that the foods you eat are actually the foods your body wants and that the movement you perform is what your body covets. You don't have to force your body to do the things that it cries out it doesn't want to do. Perhaps, just perhaps, you will eventually see the path of greatest resistance defined by the "no pain, no gain" mantra of our culture for what it is: a barrier blocking the complete integration of your mind with your body. Instead, choose the path of least resistance to unlock your innate energy and allow you access to your body's inherent wisdom. You will probably learn, as I did, that what your body wants and craves is movement. Movement unleashes your body's energy potential and enhances your understanding of what steps you must take to insure a youthful and energetic life. These are the simple truths that guide me in my quest to move effortlessly and forever—truths that are as applicable to life as they are to the arena of endurance sports within which they grew.

We Are Born to Run

No other form of movement is as natural or as beneficial as running. Take one step and you re-create an experience shared by nearly every human being since the earliest progenitors of our species took their first upright step nearly a million years ago. And what a step it was! For the first time in history, humans saw the world from eyes that gazed forward, not down. Standing on two limbs, not four, our ancestors were able to use their forelimbs and hands to carry food, forage, and care for and carry their young. Freeing of the hands led to the emergence of tool-making and the development of technology, both for hunting and agriculture. When humans began to move by supporting their weight on two legs, they developed a unique locomotion pattern that involved the rhythmic shifting of body weight. This constant one-foot-in-front-of-the-other cadence became the dance of life for our species. It was a movement form like no other, asking us to perpetually monitor and balance ourselves on the most precarious of platforms—our own two legs. Out of this constant balancing act emerged an aerobic fat-based energy metabolism that could sustain activity for longer and longer periods of time. Because of this proficient, energy-conserving metabolism, humans were able to roam far and wide, displaying hunting, gathering, and migratory skills never before seen in land-based animals. Our ancestors, if not the fastest or most powerful living land creatures, were certainly the most relentless and wide ranging.

Over the course of hundreds of thousands of years, human physiology adjusted to a life that alternated between standing, walking, running, and squatting in search of seeds, berries, grubs, insects, and other food sources. For better balance, we developed the current version of our big toe. Our shoulders became slightly smaller, the chest more streamlined, and the vast complex of muscles, tendons, and skeletal alignments shifted and adjusted to accommodate a more efficient vertical bipedal stance. Our cranial structure changed as well. The brain grew larger, creating even more balancing challenges, precariously situated on top of the vertically erect spine. These balancing challenges were answered by the emergence of the most incredible network of neuromuscular controls, which imbued us with a sense of balance and gait that enabled us to get around, survive, and flourish.

The point is that our physiology is exquisitely designed for running and walking. It is only when we move in a bipedal motion—running or walking—that we can fully understand and appreciate the messages and innate wisdom our bodies offer. Our bodies are magnificently suited to moving in the form of walking and running. To engage in this motion brings us one step closer to what we are.

Some people shrink from this experience for fear of injury. Others develop knee pain or some other muscle or joint discomfort when they do run, so they pursue alternative forms of movement such as swimming, cycling, or stair climbing, which offer no impact at all. While these other modes of exercise can be extremely beneficial, unless supplemented with walking or running, they keep you one step away from your most natural and expressive state—bipedal motion.

When you walk or run, you support your body weight against the force of gravity as it moves through time and space. As your body moves, the force of gravity travels through your body in a path that is directed down the spine and out the feet. Your body dissipates the weight of gravity's force as a lighting rod would divert the power of an electrical storm away from the building on which it is situated. When a skeletal system that is aligned and in balance combines with a muscular system that is strong and flexible, the stress and pressure of upright movement can be successfully routed down and out the body. Should a muscle-to-bone relationship go awry, it can disrupt the flow of energy through the body, leading to the collection rather than the dissipation of stress. The end result is pain or discomfort. If, as a result of the discomfort, you conclude that running isn't for you and seek out other forms of movement, you miss an opportunity to enhance the muscle-to-bone relationships that manage the flow of stress through the body.

Just suppose the pain and discomfort that you may experience after a run was not caused by the running but due to a prior imbalance or weakness in your body. In this scenario, the running merely uncovered or unmasked a condition that was lying unnoticed. Later on in this book, you will be asked to consider the possibility that there is a relationship between the health of your body and the relative strength and function of certain muscle groups. We are talking about internal organs such as your adrenal glands, small and large intestines, gall bladder, and liver (to name a few) and the impact they might have on the action of a specific muscle group, such as your quadriceps, hamstrings, psoas, or sartorious muscles. These muscles affect the health of the back, knee, hips, and even shoulders if the skeletal imbalances they create are severe enough. The organ dysfunctions themselves could have a wide variety of causes: poor nutrition, stress, emotional distress, overtraining, and too much sugar, alcohol, or caffeine. The pain or discomfort arising from an afternoon jog may be due to emotional stress or nutritional deficiency rather than the stress of running on your knees. Running in this instance merely clarifies the state your body is in by uncovering the imbalances that might lie hidden beneath the surface. When you run or walk, you provide yourself with an opportunity to get at this information so that you can explore the possibilities it offers. Other forms of movement that try to minimize the effect gravity has on the innate systems of the body may cover up any imbalances because they don't challenge the body in nearly the same way. Seize the opportunity to move bipedally and upright, supporting your body weight against the force of gravity. Explore where your body is right now and how you might be able to make it better.

This book does more than just show you how to use running and walking as a means of getting in closer touch with your body. It presents specific strategies about how to think, train, and eat so that you can create more energy, increase productivity, last longer, and be more at one with yourself and your body. Consider it an integrated guide to personal productivity that relies on a totally natural, readily accessible, and absolutely enjoyable process for creating energy. The key is training your body to rely on fat as its primary source of energy. This book will show you how to do this. You will be surprised at how easy it can be. In fact, the challenge for many is that it may be too easy—and enjoyable.

Many of the claims inside this book come from years of extensive scientific research and coaching experience. I have two master's degrees, one in social science and one in movement science, and more than twenty years of coaching and personal-training experience. For the most part, however, what you are about to read is a collection of insights and distinctions drawn from a journey through an unconventional world that can make a difference in your everyday life. I ask you to read with an open mind and have faith that in the end you'll know what is right for you when it comes across your path. Most often, what is right and true is so simple we wonder how we didn't recognize it sooner.

It is my first appointment with Carol, who appears to be in good shape, though she admits she has never exercised on a regular basis or paid much attention to her diet. A stock-broker with long hours, she wants to run in order to have more energy to get her through her day. Her main goals, she says, are to learn to run comfortably and burn fat in the process.

After a consultation in my office, we head out to run along the beach of La Jolla, where we both live. Carol is eager for me to talk about form, and I start by telling her to be conscious of her breathing—to breathe to a "ball" that I ask her to imagine exists inside of a triangle formed by her hips and belly button. As we continue along, I talk about her relationship to the ground as she moves. With each step I want her to imagine that the earth is rotating toward her and "feel" as though she's lifting her feet up just enough to let the earth pass beneath. I ask her to relax her hands, as though she's holding live butterflies inside her palms. I point out the three dimensionality of the world around us. I describe the expansiveness of the sensory-based information that surrounds and envelops her—the colors of the sky, the textures of the clouds, the scent of the flowers, and the rustling of the leaves on the trees. We continue running along at a pace that is comfortable and conversational. I am certain she is where I want her to be, moving effortlessly and burning fat.

Next, I pick up speed and ask Carol to keep up with me. I want her to be aware of how different her experience can be when she is no longer moving comfortably and burning fat but is in a more challenging and stressful sugar-burning state. Her form changes dramatically and instantaneously; from relaxed to stressful. Her face tightens and her breathing rises to her chest. As we run faster and faster, I describe to her the changes I know she is experiencing as she takes in the world. The quality of the visual information she is taking in has begun to change. Her attention is being drawn into a much narrower field of vision. She is no longer present to the vast panorama of sky, horizon, clouds, and trees. She seems to be staring at a small spot in front of her as she pants half-jokingly, "Why are you doing this to me?" We slow down, and I ask her to describe what she has just experienced.

"You made me run faster," she says.

"How do you know?" I reply.

"Because when we picked up the pace," she says, "I could feel my heart rate rise, and my only thoughts were about keeping up."

"What else?" I ask.

"Well, I heard my breathing get louder, and it felt shallower and more in my chest than in my belly. I certainly didn't feel relaxed anymore. I couldn't wait for you to tell me to slow down."

We run back to my office, and as we wrap up, I ask whether she has any questions. "I don't really have any questions right now," she tells me. "But I do have a comment," she shares. "This was not what I expected.

"I expected you to talk about running, but it wasn't really about that. I thought you'd tell me all about burning fat, but it wasn't really about that. You were telling me to move in a way so that I could connect with myself and with the world around me. The truth is, I always thought running was about seeing how fast I could run, not about using movement to connect with my body, and through my body connecting with the world all around me. You were telling me to see myself as part of the total flow of life; to understand that running and walking can be much bigger and have a greater purpose than just how quickly I can run a mile or lose some weight. Certainly running affects my fitness, my health, my weight, and how I look, yet it can be so much more. You helped me realize that moving in this way can be about being connected to my body and increasing my awareness of who I am and what it will take for me to succeed. You were also reminding me to enjoy myself so I love the experience and want to do it more."

I hope, like Carol, you have chosen to take action, move forward, and grow. Let go of your thoughts about how hard you think you have to push, how many goals you have to reach, and what you assume you have to do in order to be happy. Instead your only focus is to manage the moment you are in. In doing so, you might just go farther than you ever dreamed possible.

The gate is now open, exposing the path to how to think, train, and eat for the distance. All you need to do is take the first step and you are on your way to treating your mind and your body in a way that makes you feel strong and energetic, responsive, and positive. Not only will you astound yourself with what you will be capable of doing, but you will also feel great as you progress.

PART ONE

How to THINK for the Distance

I am absolutely certain we can all go farther, feel better, and be more productive than we ever imagined possible. But first we have to believe we can. Our attitude toward what we think is possible determines what we do. If you believe you can run a mile, you will. If you think you can't, you won't. Your mind will not let you. Your mindset creates the possibilities, dreams the dreams, and your body lives them.

As you begin this journey toward lasting change in the way you feel about your body and the possibilities available to you, start with the understanding that what you think is as important as what you do. Have you ever heard the saying, "Thoughts are physical"? If you were to come to my office, I could hook you up to a variety of biofeedback machines, and you would understand immediately why this statement could be true.

Just imagine lying down on a comfortable table, your body communicating to a variety of scientific apparatuses designed to monitor your heart rate, respiration, electrical activity in the muscles, energy in the brain, body temperature, and salinity of the skin. I talk to you in a calm and soothing voice and guide you into a state of deep relaxation. I ask you to imagine yourself at the starting line of a race. I want you to "see" the other runners surrounding you and feel the energy of anticipation build. In your mind you "hear" the starting pistol go off and imagine yourself running with the pack. You "feel" your heart rate racing, your breath speeding up, your arms pumping, and your legs flying. You begin living the race in your mind as I am monitoring your body. What is happening? The machines begin to pick up signals that your body is actually recreating the experience you are imagining. Your heartbeat quickens, and there are rises in your respiration rate, the temperature of your skin, and the amount of electrical activity in your muscles and brain. Your skin begins to perspire, and the monitors detect salt on the surface of your skin. Your body physically experiences the activity your mind is creating. Remarkable! What the mind conceives, the body achieves.

What goes on in your head is as important as how you physically train or what food strategies you employ. Mind, body, and nutrition are areas of training that you must develop and fine-tune, manage, and balance, much in the same way a master triathlete does his swimming, biking, and running. If you neglect one or two endeavors, they will come back to haunt you. Any system is only as strong as its weakest link.

Over the past twenty years, as an endurance athlete and coach, I have come to rely on a set of principles that program the mind to think about success in the long run. What makes these insights so powerful is that they affect not just running but also your whole life. Life is an endurance event. Use these principles to organize your thoughts as you relentlessly move forward with energy, enthusiasm, and a commitment to live life to the fullest.

Believe in Yourself
You Can Do More Than You Think

At the beginning of my seminars, I often start by asking everyone in the room to raise his or her hand. Everyone complies. Then I say, "Raise it higher," which everyone does. "Higher again," I call out, and again everyone in the room figures out a way to put their arms even higher in the air. Some stand up, others hop on the table or chair. Within moments the room is full of excitement and laughter as the point of this exercise hits home. "You see what just happened," I conclude. "Everyone in this room underestimated what he or she was capable of doing when I first asked you to raise your hands."

Expanding the boundaries of what you believe to be possible is critical in putting yourself in a position to go the distance and do the extraordinary. We need to stretch beyond self-imposed limitations.

It is late September 1987. I have just been hired to prepare a team of runners from a major hotel in New York for the upcoming New York City Marathon. The hotel's general manager, with support from his staff, believes participation in the marathon will build camaraderie and company spirit. A rally is held in the hotel's grand ballroom to introduce the team of twenty-seven runners to me—their coach. The ballroom is full of cheering staff. The team runs down the center aisle amidst clapping and cheering. Speeches are given. When it is over, I meet privately with the team.

"How many of you have ever run a marathon before?" I ask. One person raises his hand.

"What about twenty miles?" The same person raises his hand. No one else does.

"How about ten miles?" Still only the lone marathon veteran nods.

"What about 10K?" Nothing.

"A 5K?" Everyone raises his or her hands. Twenty-seven runners and only one had ever run more than 3.1 miles, the distance of the race sponsored earlier in the year by that same hotel.

The New York City Marathon is nine weeks away.

Everyone in the room laughs. We all share the humor in the improbability of it all. Twenty-seven crusaders about to embark on a marathon journey in a little more than two months with only one of them even remotely prepared to go. I think: "Well, there goes the deal." Sure I am hesitant. My initial reaction is, "I can't possibly train twenty-six novice runners to finish a marathon in nine weeks." It just can't be done! I might be acting irresponsibly if I take the hotel's money and bring this group to the starting line.

Then I reconsider. I believe in the human capacity to go the distance, that even the seemingly most ordinary of talents is capable of producing the most extraordinary of results. This event will surely put my belief to the test. My initial hesitancy changed to excitement. What an incredible opportunity!

So I get creative. "We are not going to train to run a marathon," I announce to the group of startled would-be marathoners. "We are going to learn how to participate in and enjoy a 26.2 mile-long street festival." From that point on it gets easier.

I need to reconceptualize what it is we are about to do. Running the entire marathon at breakneck speed is not an option for most of them. Indeed, I would not recommend that strategy for anyone save the most experienced and elite marathon runner. What we have to do is chunk-down our goal, making it monumental and manageable at the same time. I know that nine weeks isn't enough to train them in a conventional marathon-training program. And these are not people who have the luxury of endless amounts of free time to allocate to marathon preparation. I figure five to seven hours a week of training is probably more than most could commit to. Realistically, three to five was what I was going to get.

We develop a plan that consists of transforming the aid stations set up at one-mile intervals along the course into festival booths. Our objective becomes to visit each and every one of them. We plan on entering the staging ground of the event not as untested warriors going off to battle, but as youthful explorers about to journey through their first adventure. The feeling we want to create inside is one of curiosity and awe, excitement and calm, jubilation and anticipation. These seem infinitely more attractive and energizing than the emotional state of fear, anxiety, trepidation, and self-doubt.

But the most important thing I have to do is convince each and every runner that this goal is achievable. The general manager believes in me, that I can somehow miraculously get his group through the 26.2 miles of the New York City Marathon. Now I have to get the group to believe in themselves; that they can do it!

We spend time every day visualizing step-by-step what it is going to be like to do the event. I want them to have a plan in place prior to the race and I want them to "see" themselves confidently and assertively implementing the plan. Creative visualization involves constructing an image in your mind's eye of what it will be like when you reach your ultimate goal. Visualization concentrates the energy that springs from your desires and increases the likelihood that your dreams will be realized. With the vision of the future firmly embedded in your imagination, your mind will lead your body to the fulfillment of our thoughts. I share with the group an exercise that I use with clients prior to a big event.

"I want you to 'see' what it is like to enter the staging area. I want you to 'feel' how calm and excited you can be as you make your way to the starting line. I want you to 'hear' the ecstatic cheers of the crowd as you make your way through the carnival that is New York on this most magnificent of marathon days.

"But most of all," I continue, "I want you to see yourself in control, handling anything and everything that comes your way right up to the moment you see yourself crossing that finish line! The more powerfully you can envision this in your mind's eye the more likely your dream will come true."

I encourage them to stay relaxed, and to manage each moment. "Do this and you will be successful," I tell them. "Go with the flow. You can and will handle anything that comes along. You are going to be fine. I guarantee you'll be surprised about something. At the very least, you will learn something new about yourself and move one step closer to the ultimate goal of feeling great about your body and what you are capable of doing physically."

I take them through their training paces for the next nine weeks, ending with a run over the last three miles of the course a few days prior to the event. During that last run, I remind everyone to imagine that they are actually finishing the marathon. I ask them to "see" the finish line up ahead, to "hear" the crowd's roar of approval as they make their way up the last rise towards the finish, and "feel" the joy and exuberance running through their bodies as they finally cross the blue line.

All the runners buy into this strategy save one, the experienced marathoner. I guess, in the end, I am unable to reach him, and that he believes he cannot learn anything new from me. I must have nothing to teach him. Everyone else shows up, though, and goes on to successfully complete their first marathon run. As we wait in the hotel ballroom where the postrace reception is held, one by one the hotel runners come in. The smiles and the jubilation are contagious. They have all accomplished something that went way beyond what they had ever believed possible.

One of the runners sums it up beautifully: "I will never doubt myself again," she says to me. She then goes on to tell me about how much grief and nay saying her husband has given her from the moment she told him of her desire to run the marathon. "You can't do it," he provoked her. "Why waste your time? You'll only fail and feel even more miserably about yourself."

But she didn't fail. She triumphed! Her husband can never challenge her in that way again. She transformed her life because she believed in herself. And so can you.

The upside for believing in yourself and doing what you thought was impossible is it changes your life. You create a new reference point. The next time someone tells you can't do this or that, you can fire back, "I can. I have, and I will again."

Now, I'm not suggesting that anyone run a marathon on nine weeks' training, but I share this story to show you that it is possible. Whether it be your first marathon or your hundredth, whether you are interested in more energy for your life or the stamina to handle the start up of a new business venture at the age of fifty, going the distance is all about believing in yourself. Step out of the secure box in which you live and make a commitment to do something extraordinary. Don't be afraid to reach for the stars! Dream the most outrageous of dreams! All you need to do before you start is take a moment to envision where you would like to go. See yourself getting there, and feel what it is like to be there. The more you do this, the more likely you will get what you want. Yes, you can do it!

2

Treat Your Body As Your Partner

Use the opportunity physical training offers to get in touch with your body. Develop a relationship with your body. Approach exercise in the same way you would any other partner, colleague, lover, or mate. Sure, there are things you want to accomplish and feel you need. But can you create a successful relationship if all you do is force your wants and needs on your partner? Of course not! The ideal relationship is a dance, a give-and-take, not a do-as-I-say arrangement. You must get to know your partner, discover where you agree and disagree. You must communicate what you think will make you happy, but you must also look, listen, and feel for what your partner is saying. Sometimes you will agree. You will probably discover that your body actually thrives on many of your ambitions and desires; at other times you will learn it does not. The goal of this relationship is to act as one.

When I took up the triathlon in the early 1980s, it was a calculated decision. My manager and I thought it would make me more marketable. Still, it was a personal stretch. I was pretty fearful of open-water swimming. (Call it a shark pho-pho-pho phobia—there, I got it out!) Also, I did not feel comfortable barreling down a mountain at sixty miles per hour on what I considered a souped-up racing bike that maintained less than an inch of contact with the earth at any given time. But I trained for and completed both the Ironman and Ultraman (a double ironman) on the Big Island of Hawaii. I did rather well in both: seventy-third out of about thousand in the 1983 Ironman world championship and a remarkable (to me) second place finish at Ultraman two months later. However, once the events were over, I gradually abandoned the triathlon. It just didn't have the same effect as running did. Part of it was time management: getting to the pool, finding a place to ride the bike. I also did not enjoy the technological aspect of working on the bike. I felt infinitely greater pleasure directly relating through my body to the world around me. Running, I was in contact with the ground, with my body, to the world around me. The bike was a conduit, a piece of equipment that always felt foreign to me. I know that many bikers speak with great passion about the relationship they have with their bikes, the at-oneness they feel sitting on the seat, pedaling through life. But, that's just not me.

Swimming was a little different. My body certainly enjoyed swimming more than the biking, but still not as much as the running. I just do not like being cold—that much I know about my body. I still make it a rule to not travel to a cold climate voluntarily. When I vacation, I go to the beach or the dessert, never to the mountains. The only place I swim is in Hawaii, a heated pool, or the Jacuzzi. But I know now that it's not because of the sharks.

So I run. Everyday. It brings me joy and makes my body feel alive. That is me. The challenge for you is to discover what kind of movement is you. The way to do this is to move. Experiment. Try out different things. If you are afraid of a sport or distance, go to it. Something that generates a potent response must have meaning for you; it is revealing something about you and about your body. Put yourself in a position to discover a new aspect of yourself, a side of yourself you didn't know before. Participate, take action, and do something—anything! For the reasons outlined in the introduction, if you don't already run or walk, I strongly recommend that you do so, if not as your main activity, then at least as an adjunct to whatever else you do. The most important point, though, is to give yourself the opportunity to "dance with your partner." Few things in life can generate as much pleasure and joy as when two entities—especially the mind and body—join together and move as one.

3

Be the Master of Your Own Fate

In this age of information overload, the question that gets asked most often is, "Which expert is right?" The search goes on for the trainer with the secret program, the nutritionist with the newest angle, or the coach with the greatest track record. Should you work out harder in less time, or is it better to take it easy and aim for a longer training session? How often do you need to exercise, and what type of exercise is best? The same goes with respect to choosing what foods to eat. Do you choose high-carbohydrate and low-fat diet or a high-protein and low-carbohydrate one? Can you drink milk? What about artificial sweeteners, are they okay? And on and on . . .

With so many experts and so many opinions, many people end up concluding that the experts themselves don't know what they are talking about. This can get especially emotionally charged if you follow a path set out by an expert who doesn't lead to any noticeable results. Then the temptation is to blame the expert and the information he presents. The truth is that the expert might be right for others, but his message might not be right for you. Blaming the expert is of no consequence. What can be is accepting the fact that you and you alone are responsible for your own fate. You must always participate in the decisions that affect your life, your body, your energy, and your health. There is no expert alive—no physician, nutritionist, or personal trainer—who can take your place when it comes to making the decisions about your body that really matter.

Shifting the focus from the experts to you makes you the center of attention. The expert that's right for you is you. It's the person in the mirror. The direction of your path is to not focus on the expert but to focus on yourself. In order to discover what's best for you, you must learn to be in touch with your body and capable of processing the information your body sends you. The challenge is to be constantly aware of what is going on in your body and being educated about what is current in the world of health of fitness. This doesn't mean you must be an expert in the minutiae of current scientific research. That is where experts can come in—not to tell you what to do, but to inform you of your options so you can make the most informed decisions. You must, though, be able to ask the right questions of your body and the health practitioners with whom you choose to work.

If you are striving for consistent energy and enthusiasm about your physical program, bear in mind that these are the kinds of questions you need to ask in order to discover whether or not the course of action you have chosen is working for you.

- Do you wake up fatigued or tired?
- Does your energy level fluctuate over the course of the day?
- Do you need to eat to get energy?
- Do you lose energy between meals, especially after high-carbohydrate or sugar-filled ones?
- Do you have difficulty concentrating or thinking clearly?
- Are you moody, irritable, or depressed?

Unless you answer "no" to all of these questions, you need to adjust your strategies. As you will see later, in the training and nutrition sections, common causes of inconsistent energy and fatigue are diets high in sugar, an overreliance on caffeine, and a training program dependent on anaerobic, sugar-burning exercise. Your main objective is to raise your level of awareness about who you are and how your body works. You want to learn what kind of foods energize you, bring you pleasure, and keep you healthy and free of colds, flus, and allergies. What activities do you look forward to that make you feel youthful, vibrant, and full of life? The journey of a lifetime does not begin by choosing a course of action out of fear, believing that you should lose weight because everyone tells you to, or thinking that running a fast marathon time will make you a better person. These are disempowering mindsets.

An empowering one is driven by the excitement of self-discovery. It steers you along the path of possibilities and encourages you to become present to and participate in the creation of your future life. It must start with the premise that no matter how learned and well versed the experts are, you and only you can, in the end, be the master of your own fate. Who is in the position and has the capacity to know you better than you? No one! Too many of us get led astray by false fitness prophets who are only out to impress us with how much they know. Or, worse yet, how much better they know than we do what is good for us. It's not about the experts—it's about you! You and your well-being are at stake, not the reputation and credentials of the experts you consult. Keep that in mind as you take the next step of your lifelong journey.

There will be times when you will face a clear-cut fork in the road: an expert will say go one way, and your body will say go the other. These are the moments when a breakthrough is possible. Which way do you go? How strong is the connection you have with your body? Do you have faith in yourself? Do you have the courage to act on what feels right to your body, as opposed to what an expert says?

When your body tells you something, you have an opportunity. If you seize that opportunity, you will move one step closer to being the master of your own fate. Even if you are wrong, you will have learned something. More than likely, though, you will be right. And if you have the faith and courage to act on it, in spite of what someone else might be telling you, you begin to control your own destiny and increase the likelihood that you will be successful in the your lifelong journey.

It is 1993, and I am at a seminar in Cancun, Mexico. I am with a client named Peggy, circling a track alongside the ocean in the midday heat. We have been moving for nearly an hour, shifting from running to walking and back again. Peggy is wearing a heartrate monitor transmitter belt, and I am checking her heartrate with the receiver I have strapped to my wrist. We are trying to set an ideal target zone for her to train in. We crisscross the target-zone setting a number of times, and I check how she is doing. I encourage her to stay in touch with her experience. I want her to breathe comfortably—low to the belly, without the noticeable forced expulsion of air that signifies the effort is getting too hard and she is moving into a stressful sugar-burning state. I coach her on how to position her arms, how to relate to the ground with her feet, and where to look and how to "see" with her eyes. She is flowing now, moving effortlessly, comfortably. I can tell. She is smiling. Her body is calm and relaxed. Her movement is silent. I turn to her and say, "You're there! Perfect! Just stay where you are and you will be in the perfect place to begin your program."

Peggy gives me a pondering look. She stops, puts her hands to her face and begins to sob.

Now I have no idea what is happening. I put my arm around her and ask her if she is okay. She begins to calm down, and with tears still moving down her face she looks up at me and smiles.

"I always enjoyed moving like this," she says. "But my friends all told me I was not working hard enough to get anywhere. So I pushed myself harder and harder, and never enjoyed it anymore. I eventually stopped walking and running because I grew to hate it. Now you are saying that all along I was doing what was right for me. I am crying because you gave me my experience back. Thank you."

Peggy was listening to her body and enjoying the experience she had as she moved. Her friends told her she had to work harder, though, and she began listening to her friends, not her body. In so doing, Peggy lost out on an opportunity to explore who she was, what her body wanted, and instead settled for discovering how much pain she could take. I call this the electric-socket theory of training. Each day becomes a test to see how much current your body can take when you plug your finger into the outlet. All you ever discover with this how-much-can-you-take mentality is the strength of the current that breaks you down.

Peggy has a much nobler goal in mind. She is now asking, "What can I do today that brings me joy and makes me feel good about my body and my life?" Putting herself through pain and misery just isn't one of those things.

Now Peggy's friends might not necessarily qualify as "experts" in the true sense of the word. Yes, we all are influenced by a variety of people, hawking their goods at the expense of our own sense of what seems to be right for us. Some are subtle, some less so. There are doctors, coaches, parents, nutritionists, and fitness gurus galore spewing forth contrasting and competing opinions on how to maximize energy, lose weight, and live forever. The health and fitness world is jam-packed with opposing belief systems, ambitious one-of-a-kind programs, and self-assured authorities who have discovered the magic formula of the month for immediate and long-lasting results. There are proponents of vegetarianism, food combining, and high protein; there are advocates of weightlifting, running, swimming, and cross training. All are true believers; all have followers; all have the requisite backlog of testimonials. Yet "all" may not be right for you. Only one might be, or a combination of a few of them, or the strategy of someone you have not discovered yet. The only empowering question is not which one of them is right, but which one is right for you!

What I am proposing to you is that committing to being physical, taking action, and doing something with your life carry a burden of responsibility. You are responsible for your own fate. You must be involved in the decisions that shape and influence your life. Just following what some expert says is right may not be what is in your best interest. There are no graded report cards in the classroom of your life. You are not graded *A* to *F* on how well you follow the program the expert designs for you. Getting an *A* on following instructions means nothing if the strategy you employ doesn't make sense for you.

This path isn't necessarily easy. There are times when I also would prefer just to have someone tell me what to do. I remember a well-known runner on the comeback trail telling me he'd made a name for himself as a sponsored athlete for a major company. Now, after years of not competing, he said all he needed to do was to get back with his coach, follow the old program, and he'd be on top again. To me, that's an oversimplification of what it's all about. Life goes on, things change. What worked then may not work now. We are not mass-produced machines coming off of an assembly line with an operator's manual that works equally well for all of us.

There's a great part of the population base just now coming into health and fitness with an eagerness to learn and a commitment to change. They are showing up because they are concerned about health later in life. They also are coming in open-minded and in need of a coach they can trust. With most of these people, almost any change will create a positive benefit. Say you've been existing on a diet of fast food, coffee, and cocktails and haven't been feeling your best. At your annual check up, your doctor warns you that you need to improve your diet. Well, if you eat nothing but pears, there'll be a positive benefit. But can you exist on pears the rest of your life? Either consciously or unconsciously, you can't survive on pears. Which way do you go? Many people bounce from program to program. I hear, "I have a nutritionist who sent me to a lymph specialist who said I shouldn't eat meat, and now I'm on forty–thirty–thirty diet." What I hear are people who speak through the people they see. I try to get people to talk about their own experiences.

The idea that someone outside of you could have the answers to all your questions is an impossibility. Who can know you better than yourself? You are the captain of your own ship, the master of your own destiny. You must come up with your own plan based upon the information you have and take responsibility for the results you get.

I for one will not give up the power to decide what is best for my body. I hope you will take charge of your life and do the same. No one knows you better than you do. This is not to say that you or I know more about muscle testing, massage, acupuncture, or conventional medicine than the experts who are trained in those fields. But I do know more about myself, and you about yourself. While you and I can value their input, we have to make day-to-day decisions about our bodies that are based on what we perceive to be in our best interests. These experts can have input; we must have the final say.

4

Stay in the Moment—the Future Will Take Care of Itself

The successful endurance athlete must make peace with the infinitude of time. Time is everlasting. We are but a moment in time, yet we are permanently and everlastingly linked to its eternal essence. It is only when we allow ourselves to accept this that we will truly succeed.

This mindset is much different than that of the sprinter, who wants to get there as quickly as possible. Our objective is to be part of time, revel in its abundance, and be open to its wisdom. We must move away from the belief that time is scarce and that getting through time is of maximum importance. Let go of the idea that the first one who gets there wins. Says who? What if getting there is not really all that important and being here is?

A fixation on getting through time demeans the experiential here-and-now. It renders the moments we live less important than the place we want to go. There is no good reason to rush through time in a mad dash to get to where you want to go. Everything is all around you; everything is here; time is abundant and time is precious. Savor each moment. Open yourself up to the lessons you might learn along the way.

When I race, I never run to a finish line. I immerse myself in the moment I am living. With every step, I access where I am in my breathing cycle. I feel my body making contact with the ground. I adjust my arm position, my pace. My mantra is, "Manage the moment."

Success in the thousand-mile race of life is no different. Being "here" is the most important thing. The "there" will come; it always does. Make the most of the now. Embrace it. Keep yourself open to the possibilities your immersion into the moment may bring.

It is the tenth day of the thousand-mile race. Sigfried Bauer, the current world-record holder, has just walked off the track. I am alone now, just me and the distance. We have been battling for hours through the night, each of us determined to stay on the track at all costs. We both believe that whoever walks off first will be conceding the race to the other. I am more than thirty miles ahead at the time. Sigfried finally breaks, stops running, and leaves the track. He ends up staying in his tent for more than four hours. The race is now over. I am certain I will win and set a new world record. Soon the excitement of the hunt wanes. The hours that had flown by earlier in the heat of the battle now slow to a painful standstill. I still have more than a full day to go before the event will end. I start to struggle, more mentally than physically. A runner joins me. It is Marvin Skaggerberg, a veteran of the Bunion Derby, a trans-America road race that was held earlier in the year. Marvin asks me how I am doing. I am having a rough time getting myself going, my tank is near empty, and I feel confused and strangely detached from what is going on around me. I look at Marvin and say, "I don't know. It just seems as if this thing is just never going to end."

Marvin smiles the wisdom of a man who has just run

3,600 miles. "Stu," he replies, "the one thing you have to accept is that they always do . . . they always do. The race is what it is. The future will take care of itself. Your job is to take care of this moment."

There's no real upside to trying to control time and focus on when the end will come. As Marvin reminded me, the end always will come. Don't rush it. Be present to the passing of time.

Body-Awareness Exercise—How to Be "Here" Now

Focus on your breathing.

Imagine a triangle formed by your hips and belly button. Inside of the triangle is a "ball." As you breathe in, fill the "ball" up with air. Feel the "ball" expand as you breathe in, and "feel" the air coming out of the ball as you breathe out. Inhale to the count of four, hold to the count of eight, and exhale to the count of six.

Assess your relationship to the ground.

Stand up. Feel your body weight being supported by your feet. Let your arms hang comfortably by your side, and evenly distribute your weight on each foot. Bend your knees slightly, and shift your weight back so that your body weight is being almost entirely supported by your heels. Wiggle your toes. Notice how stable and relaxed you feel. Now shift your weight forward so you end up on your tiptoes. Your weight is now being borne by the front of your foot. Notice the difference in how you feel. In which stance were you more stable and relaxed, and in which one were you more tense and unstable?

Observe your surroundings.

How does the world look? Notice its depth and colors. Take in as much information as you can. How many different colors can you see? Listen for sounds, nearby and far away. Can you make out three distinct sounds? How about four? Five? Breathe and be aware of the different fragrances that surround you. What do they remind you of? How do they make you feel?

Take a mental inventory of your body.

If you find an area that's more tense than another, imagine your breath filling up the area and relaxing it. Release all tension as you exhale. Note the fluidity and warmth as your body continues to move. Play with your arm position. Check the tension in your hands and in your jaw. Relax.

5

Set Process-Oriented Goals

Occasionally I meet people whose happiness is dependent on a future outcome. Some are certain that their life will change and they will be happy if only they could run a three-hour marathon. To others, it is a "knock 'em dead, not-an-ounce-of-body-fat body" or making a million dollars or buying the house they've always wanted. But I ask you the same question I ask my clients: Have you ever known someone who reached his or her marathon time goal, had a great body, or had money and a house who felt neither happy nor fulfilled? I have, and I am sure many of you have also. What we accomplish is not who we are. The awards and achievements are ornaments on the tree but do not necessarily define who we are and what possibilities exist. If you are happy with who you are, all of these "ornaments" can be quite enjoyable; if you are not, they will bring you nothing more than momentary amusement.

Not only have I known people like this, I was once one of them. I, too, was susceptible to defining my worth by how successfully I performed. If only I could do well in a triathlon, if only I could win this race, if only I could set a world record, if only I could reach my late forties with a body like the one I had in my early twenties, I would be happy. I've been there, done that. And each time I got there, something else came up that seemed to get in the way of my truly being at peace with myself, with being happy, feeling worthy. Oh, it's nice to have people be impressed with what you've done. But if you are dependent upon the accolades of others to confer value on your life, you give up whatever power you have to create your own meanings in life.

What about the people who run from one "if-only-I-could-do-this" goal to the next, seeking that one breakthrough achievement that will bring them eternal happiness? It might happen. I haven't seen it yet. The most powerful transformation came when I knew someone who went into an event with one set of goals and emerged with another.

When I first meet Thomas, a business owner and family man, he had already completed a marathon. It was one of a long list of goals he wished to accomplish. He followed the prescribed marathon-training plan from a running magazine and completed the Marine Corps Marathon. Then it was on to the next goal (definitely not another marathon).

When he comes to see me, he no longer enjoys running, describing it as "grueling" and "a test of fortitude." He just can't get past three miles in his training, but he wants to continue running to keep his weight down and to alleviate stress.

After a series of sessions, Thomas slowly shifts his focus from time and distance goals to the process of running. He starts focusing on how he feels as he runs, and with some minor adjustments discovers that he can actually "enjoy" the process of running. He's running more slowly than before, but that doesn't matter to him right now, because he is actually beginning to look forward to each movement session. Anyway, I convince him that the speed at which he runs does change, and in time he will probably speed up without even working any harder. What is important now is that he feel comfortable as he moves. As if by magic, his miles gradually pick up and so does his time. By running within his target heart-rate zone, his headaches go away. He sets a new goal: to run forever. By changing his focus, Thomas accesses a world that was once closed to him because his sights were set not on enhancing the quality of his experience but on evaluating the significance of the outcome.

When we focus more on the process than the outcome, we realize that true empowerment does not exist in the goals that lie outside of our body. True empowerment comes from waking up each and every morning and thinking, moving, and eating in ways that give us energy and allow total integration in a life mission that instills passion and generates a life we love.

Keep your mind focused on the process. You will discover that a process orientation allows more room to be creative, have fun, handle adversity, and adjust to life's inevitable twists and turns. Instead of being self-absorbed with the future, cultivate a process-oriented mindset, and replace outcome goals with process-oriented ones.

Examples of process goals include the following:

- Wake up with a smile.
- Start each day acknowledging how happy you are to be alive.
- Incorporate time for movement every day.
- Drink plenty of water.
- Eat a balanced, healthy diet.
- Be vigilant in accessing the experience you are having.
- Interact and have fun with the people around you.

These are standards that you can regularly meet, and they increase the likelihood that your day-to-day objectives will be realized. Nothing ensures success better than success. Each successful day brings you closer to your goal of optimal health and moving through life with genuine satisfaction and happiness. Learn to stay focused on the process:

- Be aware of where you are in the breathing cycle.
- Let results emerge gradually—don't force things!
- Focus on the experience you are having, not on the results you want later.
- It's not about how much you're doing, it's about how well you are experiencing it.
- Focus on comfort and joy, not on pain and discomfort.
- Be positive, stay present—the future is yet to come and still remains under your control.
- The more you focus on the process, the faster the results will come.

6

Move Forward in Small, Manageable Increments

Remarkably, huge distances such as fifty miles, a hundred miles, or even a thousand miles don't overwhelm the seasoned endurance athlete. The secret lies in breaking down enormous tasks into manageable segments. We complete an increment and move on. Then we complete another one, rest, and move on yet again and again and again. The key to success lies in creating a succession of little victories, each one empowering the next.

When time came for me to challenge the thousand-mile distance, I did not take on the task of running a thousand miles. I committed myself to running one mile one thousand times. Running a thousand miles was too far beyond my ability to comprehend, like a trillion dollars. I know what the words say, but I can't really comprehend what they mean.

There is magic in creating a structure that guides you toward a productive and infinitely manageable state and away from overextending yourself to the point where you'll need too much time to recover. This is the heart of endurance—it is not an attempt to discover how much pain and discomfort we can take before we break down and need to recover. Endurance isn't about achieving and holding on to a stressful state for as long as you can. Quite the opposite. Optimizing productivity for a prolonged period requires that you maintain a much more manageable state over smaller repeatable increments.

It is 1983, and Fred Lebow, the president of the New York Road Runners Club, is putting together a six-day race of historical significance. Six-day events are starting to reemerge after nearly a century of neglect. The six-day, go-as-you-please foot races originally appeared in the 1880s and left an indelible mark in the running world by setting running records that remained unchallenged to that very day. Six-day races were designed to provide an opportunity for the contestants to discover how many miles they could cover in six consecutive days. The go-as-you-please moniker pertained to the fact that participants were free to walk, run, jog, or skip—whatever it took to keep moving forward. The six-day time frame emerged because there were laws against public congregation on the Sabbath back then, so the race began at midnight Sunday and ended on midnight Saturday. The other intriguing aspect is that the events generated a lot of money and interest, two factors that of which Fred and the participants were keenly aware.

Fred decides to resuscitate this monster event by inviting every internationally renowned multiday running star to his event, which is slated to begin on July 4, 1983.

Although I have been vaguely aware of Fred's intentions, I let this awareness slide into the remote regions of my consciousness because I am so intent on competing in the hundred-miler scheduled a month earlier. There is no way I can do both events. Besides, I am not a multiday runner. I've never run more than twenty-four hours at a time. I am a hundred-mile specialist.

As fate would have it, thirteen miles into the hundred-mile race I am hit by a bike and eventually drop out of the event at around the 50-mile mark. Eager for a new challenge and to ease the disappointment of a DNF (did not finish) next to my name, I give Fred a call and request to be allowed in to the six-day race. He welcomes me in the event. He even hooks me up with ABC News *NightLine*, which arranges to have me report each night to Ted Koppel and inform a national network audience what it's like to run around a track for six consecutive days on less than four hours of sleep a day.

I have a plan, or think I do, which, I guess, is the point of this story. My plan is simple. I'll start the race and run until I can't run anymore. Then I'll stop and rest. Once rested, I'll run some more, until I no longer feel like running again, at which point I'll rest yet again, repeating the pattern until the race is over. That was my plan. Probably not that dissimilar from the plan by which I had been living my life at the time. And it works . . .

. . . for a while, but . . .

. . . by day two, after about thirty-six hours of all running and no sleep, I am totally out of it. Burnt. Nothing left in the tank. Not even the promise of a Ted Koppel *NightLine* interview with ABC network news can get me out of my funk. As the second night drags on, I struggle mightily. I hobble one quarter of the way around the quarter-mile track, walk to the side, and lie down to nap for a few minutes. I get up and wander around the track again, maybe covering the entire quarter mile. Exhausted, I go to my tent and rest, hoping for rejuvenation, which never comes. I head back to the track, run a bit more, and on it goes. As dawn approaches, I become aware that over the past seven hours I have managed to cover a measly five miles—just twenty laps of the quarter mile all-weather track! I am devastated, confused, and ready to drop out.

Nathan, a fellow ultra runner who has known me for nearly five years, observes my beleaguered state and joins me as I struggle to complete another lap. Nathan holds a very special place in the ultra community; he's considered the poet laureate of the running world. He has the keen eye and verbal ability to capture and communicate the essence of the "run." He is tall and lanky, with a scraggly gray beard and matching hair. He wears a variety of headgear, ranging from baseball cap to straw beach hat. And depending on the time of day, he dons a different pair of cut-off blue jeans in a variety of lengths, and changes from a long-sleeved plaid shirt to a white button-down cotton or short-sleeved tie-dyed T-shirt.

As we continue circling the track, Nathan puts his arm around my shoulder and begins to talk to me. "I have been watching you wander aimlessly around this track for nearly half a day now," Nathan says. "You have no rhyme or reason to your movements; no rhythm to your day." He suggests I watch the other, more experienced multiday runners and asks me what I see. The mere fact that Nathan is talking to me and getting my mind off of how tired and miserable I feel is a momentary blessing. I don't know what he is getting at. I shrug my shoulders and mumble something like, "They seem to be moving, and I'm not."

"They have a pattern, a structure to their day," he reasons. The concept is so simple and powerful at the same time. I am immediately attracted to it. "Look at Ziggy over there," Nathan motions with his arm.

The "Ziggy" Nathan is referring to is Sigfried Bauer of New Zealand. Ziggy is one of the most feared and respected of all the multiday runners. He would be the eventual winner of this first NYRRC six-day race. Ziggy's and my paths would eventually cross a number of times. It is Ziggy's thousand-mile world record I would eventually break, in a race in which he would participate and come in second.

"Ziggy just doesn't get up and run till he can't run anymore. He creates a pattern, and then repeats the pattern throughout the day," Nathan explains. "For Ziggy, it is four-and-a-half hours of relatively strong running followed by a thirty-minute break. Once the break is over, Ziggy gets back on track and powers through his next four-and-a-half hour segment.

"Ziggy never lets himself get to the point where he can't go anymore. He always takes a scheduled break prior to that point. He remains in control, making the decision. He isn't waiting for his body to break down and his energy to deplete before getting his rest. That way he is always in a position to be productive."

I take a moment to pay attention to what Ziggy is doing. The momentum and energy created by successfully reaching each incremental goal is noticeable and seductive.

Nathan and I continue circling the track as the hot humid July day begins to close in and soak through us. We analyze the other patterns the more experienced runners seem to develop. Nathan turns to me and offers, "You too must create a structure for your day.

"Create a doable and repeatable pattern right away, before this event slips away totally," he reminds me. "It doesn't have to be much. Try jogging each straightaway and walking the turns for one hour. Then take a break. Then walk a mile, run a mile. It doesn't matter as long as you set a pattern that can be repeated."

I heed Nathan's advice and begin to reorganize my race. Soon a rhythm and structure begin to set in. I am not running for four more days. I am completing the next segment. I realize that the patterns I establish are not challenging enough, so I experiment and extend them for longer and longer stretches. I soon discover that I seem to thrive on a six-hour repeatable segment. I am aware that I am running more slowly than Ziggy but am able to handle it for longer periods of time. I also notice that I only need twenty minutes for my break, the extra ten minutes doesn't seem to make that much of a difference in terms of how productive I am during the ensuing running segment.

My race slowly but surely comes together at a time when some of the other runners' races begin to unravel. I begin to move up the field. On day three, I run more miles than anyone else, an achievement I repeat on days four and six. In the end, I place second out of thirty-four of the greatest multiday runners in the world, and I set a new modern-day American record of 488 miles over six days. I learn the value of generating a plan around a repeatable pattern. This lesson has been so important in my life; I offer it to you.

Use Aid Stations to Recharge

The main challenge in building your repeatable pattern is to build in rest and recovery stages that can be taken voluntarily, before they are absolutely necessary. You can then resume the pattern again with a continued sense of accomplishment, rhythm, and flow. The beauty of this strategy is that you begin to associate productive time with positive integration, being in control, and keeping things manageable and in perspective. Your productive phase never gets out of hand or becomes something you want to avoid.

Conceive of each day as a stretch of road with aid stations every mile. What do you want to drink and eat? How much will you walk? The aid stations can act as an oasis where you can reorganize and regroup.

During seminars I meet with clients in nonstop ninety-minute increments, from 5:30 A.M. to 7:30 P.M. My pattern is to create an "aid station" after each client. I walk around the room, eat a few almonds, and drink water. I use the restroom. I don't drink any coffee or eat anything with sugar during this time. After each break I am back into a positive state. In my line of work, the first portion of what I do with each client is the same, so I can establish a sense of rhythm to the session and to the day. Over time I've come to understand how many people I can handle. I've found a pattern that works for me. The day moves quickly in a pattern. Instead of seven appointments I have five left, then three. By 7:30, I shower and leave the room with a tremendous sense of accomplishment.

Whenever you are organizing an event of marathon proportions, the scale of the task can be overwhelming. If there is no point of reference, then you have no means of creating an accessible and manageable feel for what is in store and how you will be able to handle it. Some people simply throw caution to the wind and take off, believing that through the pain and suffering a new and more remarkable person will emerge. But it rarely works that way, unless the pain and suffering is what you want.

There is a way to transform the most unfathomable challenge into a repeatable series of manageable journeys. We can adapt to anything if we make the right demands on ourselves. The key is to do this incrementally—little by little. In order to make the extraordinary a reality, you must start with a plan designed to get you to your goals one step at a time.

7

Have the Courage to Stick with Your Plan

As you embark on the endurance training program, most all of the time you will be working and performing at a level of intensity far below an all-out teeth-grinding, chest-popping, and muscle-quivering maximal effort. You will, by design, be holding back, moving in a comfortable zone that you can manage and handle. There will be no on-the-brink-of-exhaustion triumph of mind over matter—just the natural unfolding of a well-conceived and eminently doable plan. This could be an affront to a culture steeped in the macho jock notion that only when you hurt can you make progress.

Be forewarned: the adjustment is as much mental as it is physical. As people switch over from a speed to an endurance mindset, one of the main challenges has to do with ego. Running within a comfort zone defined by a target heart rate means that at first you'll probably be moving much more slowly than before. You may end up running faster, but that probably won't be the case at the start. By allowing your body to start out more slowly in the zones, you will learn to become more productive in them and eventually speed up.

I receive a call from a new client, Wesley, an aggressive businessman. He expresses concern that after all his years running he now finds it disconcerting to run so slowly. Teenage girls and grandmothers are regularly passing him by. Wesley's pride is hurt; his ego bruised. I asked him how his body actually feels when he is running so comfortably and what his energy levels are like after he runs. He says he feels great, has plenty of energy, and has noticed that his ability to concentrate and remain focused is improving. Yet, regardless of the fact that his body likes training in the slower, more comfortable zones, and his mental acuity seems to be getting better, his mind needs to think he is better than the other runners. I point out that he is reacting more to his thoughts about what he "thinks" and how he "looks" than to his body's feelings about what he is actually experiencing.

I encourage Wesley to stick with his program, and remind him that he'll probably speed up eventually. In the meantime, he needs to stay present to his body.

In sports and in life, too many factors are outside of our control. The only thing we can control is the action we take. A long-term strategy will lead you toward ultimate success. Keep showing up. Stay present. Stick to the plan.

It is now 1984, and I have been working with my new trainer, Phil Maffetone, for just one week. He suggests an alternative way of preparing for the upcoming six-day world championship in La Rochelle, France. Rather than trying to run the entire distance, he wants me to divide my time between walking and running. I am not excited about this strategy. It is sacrilegious to me, although many of the original go-as-you-please contestants of the late 1880s were able to routinely average more than ninety miles a day, dividing their time between walking and running. The difference between what they did then and what

Phil was proposing to me now had to do with how the event would be laid out, so to speak.

One hundred years ago multiday runners would pile up enormous mile totals early in the event and then hang on for dear life. It was not unusual for six-day race competitors to average more than a hundred miles a day for the first two days and have their mile totals drop into seventy-mile range—even down into the sixties—as the race wore one. Phil suggests that I attempt to organize the event more evenly, that my daily average be relatively the same each day. Now I don't have too much of a problem with that since my racing style was already moving in that direction. I had even put together a six-day performance that was a negative split, meaning that I covered more miles in the last three days than I did during the first three. What I do have a problem with is Phil's intention of putting together a plan that has me, by design, walking for extended periods. That bugs me, and I tell him so. He manages to convince me otherwise and we set out to finalize the plan.

I will walk for the entire first hour of each five-hour segment. The next hour I will run, followed by another one-hour walk, another one-hour run, and finishing with a third and final one-hour walk. The plan projects me walking at fifteen minutes a mile, or four miles an hour. I would run at an eight minutes-per-mile clip, or exactly 7.5 miles per hour. This plan called for me to cover twenty-seven miles during each five-hour segment, enabling me to complete nearly four of these sequences each day.

I arrive in La Rochelle. The race is held in an exposition hall, just outside the castle walls. Thousands of people arrive for the opening ceremonies. We are introduced to the loyal spectators. Many of them already know about us or have met us during the many scheduled visits we have made to the local homes, schools, and businesses. The crowd cheers each and every runner, yet I feel a special response when I am introduced. Not for me per se, but for the fact that I am the only American in a World Championship event attended by a swarm of people that seemed madly infatuated by anything American.

Amidst this incredible scene and amongst people I want so much to please, I am beginning to get jittery and faint hearted. What is happening? I am having second thoughts about my plan to start the event walking.

The event begins, and the runners are off. The crowd roars and the music blares thunderously on. What do I do? I start walking. The crowd begins to yell, but not in support. I manage to hear taunts of "Yankee, go home!" mixed in with the more universal and easy to understand "boo."

By the end of the first hour, I am in dead last out of a field of more than twenty invited runners. Then I start my run. Now I move back up the field, only to fall back once again when my walk period recommences. This pattern plays out over the next two days. Back and forth, up and down. I end up somewhere in the bottom third of the field at the end of day two.

On day three, I am sticking to my plan, fifteen-minutes-a-mile walking, followed by eight-minutes-a-mile running. It is becoming noticeable to the spectators that I am running more powerfully than just about anyone else in the race. Even when I walk, I am still moving faster than some of the other contestants are running. I am getting stronger while everyone else is weakening. By the end of day four, I am now closing in on the two leaders, Jean-Gils Boussiquet and his younger protégé, Patrick Simmonet. I have made up nearly fifty miles over the past three days and am now just behind Patrick and within thirty miles of Jean-Gils. The crowd is absolutely with me by this point. It is remarkable. "Allez Mittleman! Allez." "Go, Mittleman, Go!" I notice Patrick begins to change his race strategy to respond to what I am doing. It is something I remember for a later time. For in this most extraordinary of racing formats, the competitors aren't running against each other, but against each other's routines. Which competitor's routine will produce the most miles? The one who just tries to run the whole time, or the one with a plan? For the moment, it seems that the one with the plan is in control.

As day six begins I am now just twenty miles behind Jean-Gils, and the same distance ahead of Patrick. I chase Jean-Gils over the course of the next eighteen hours. True champion that he is, Jean-Gils rallies and maintains his lead to the very end. With four hours left, he turns to me and whispers, "ce n'est possible,"—it is not possible. We have reached that moment of mutual recognition and relief, when there is no time left to alter the inevitable.

With just four hours remaining, there is not enough time to make up the twenty miles, as long as Jean-Gils remains on the track, which he has shown he is able to do. Anyway, at that time it is challenging enough just to run twenty miles in four hours without trying to catch someone. It is over, I agree. We hug and help each other through the end of the event.

I have made my mark, though. One of the La Rochellais approaches me after the closing ceremonies. I have been aware of him throughout the event. He sat in the same spot every night, with a stopwatch in hand, recording lap after lap of the lead runners. He, more than anyone there, seemed to both understand and savor the inner dynamics of the multi-day race. "I have never seen a race like that before," he manages to communicate to me. "Bravo, Mittleman."

What about you? What is your long-term plan? Remind yourself at every turn that the decisions you make must benefit you not just today but tomorrow and the next day and the next. Surround yourself with people who will support you on your long-term mission. Last, but not least, you must realize that in order to realize fully the power of the plan, you must have the flexibility to change the plan when it isn't working.

8

Act As If Everything That Happens Is for the Good

No matter what happens in your life, everything is for the good. You must believe that. It is the most powerful, life-transforming mindset you can adopt. There is a magical aspect to our lives that can only be understood if we abandon the notions of "failure" or "defeat" in the conventional sense. When something goes wrong or doesn't work, it does not have to mean you "failed." An outcome other than the one you expected could be a window of opportunity, a signpost along the journey of your life that offers a path to future greatness. For it is only when things don't go as planned that we are presented with the opportunity to change what we are doing and continue to transform. If things always worked, there would be no mandate for change, we would always stay the same. Tony Robbins has a wonderful way of expressing this. One of his favorite sayings is: "The sign of greatness can be found in how one deals with the unexpected."

Early in my running career, I framed my assessment of what I did in terms of winning or losing: I either had a winning effort or a losing one. I could only evaluate what I did in terms of whether I did it better than someone else or my own past performances. I was so intent on how I did, I never really considered who I was; I didn't look at what I was doing in terms of the impact it had on me as a person. Just what are the lessons I am learning? Am I becoming the kind of person I want to be around? Or am I just narrowing the focus of my life to just a single, controllable variable, doomed for the rest of my life to pester others and bore myself with either running stories or injury reports? The answers become clear the moment I start changing my perspective.

Everything you do is "good," as is everything that happens to you. You don't win or lose, you only choose to grow, gain power, and flourish as a person, or not. Who you are, the kind of person you become, emerges out of how you respond to the events that happen in your life. How well you perform has little to do with it. The only real meaning derives from how you decide to "be" as a result of how things "are"—and whether you decide to move forward and try to do something about it.

It is April 1977, I arrive in Boston about to embark on a journey over the most fabled 26.2 miles in the world of running, the Boston Marathon. This is a dream come true, and a New Year's resolution fulfilled.

On January 1 of that year, I ran up Flagstaff Mountain in Boulder, Colorado. As I ascended to the top of this popular runners' path, I gazed down at the city below. It was early New Year's morning. I had the feeling that at that moment I alone was present to the world. I was happy; I felt powerful; I wanted to run a marathon. Not just any marathon, I wanted to run the Boston Marathon.

My first memory of Boston dated back to my childhood, when, as a young boy, my uncle Herbie introduced me to a training buddy of his who had done the Boston Marathon. He immediately became my childhood idol, right there alongside Mickey Mantle and Jimmy Brown. I knew then that someday I, too, would like to do that.

I ran down Flagstaff Mountain right into Frank Shorter's store. "How do I get into this year's Boston Marathon," I asked one of the salespeople stuck in the store on New Year's day. The race was in three months. "You have to qualify," he said. Back then, only runners who could break three hours (6:52 per mile) were allowed in the race. He told me the next race was the Mission Bay Marathon in San Diego. So I went and qualified, in 2 hours and 46 minutes (6:20 per mile). Then I thought what most people I know think after completing their first marathon. "My God, if I could run this well with only two weeks of preparation, imagine how much better I will do when I have two-and-a-half months to prepare—never mind taking into consideration the added experience of having done one before."

So here I am, entering the staging area in Hopkington, Massachusetts, preparing to run the race I had been dreaming about and stoked with the confidence that ten weeks of single-minded totally fanatical training brings. I organized my entire life around my Boston Marathon preparation. I cut back on my work hours, lived like an ascetic monk, trained like a maniac, ate only what *Runner's World* told me I should, and did a carbohydrate depletion followed by a carbo load in the last few days before the event. I read every book I could find on the Boston Marathon and steep myself in its tradition and lore. I wanted to be the boy in the Hans Christian Anderson fairy tale who puts on the wooden skates and comes out of nowhere to win the race.

I start making my way to the starting line. With a number in the 1900s pinned to my racing singlet, I am not able to even glimpse the starting line. How can I win the race if I have to start so far in the back of the lead pack! I formulate a plan. I notice that alongside the road is an open drainage ditch that runs parallel to the course for as far as I can see. I stand in what amounts to a long trench and begin to inch my way forward to the front. By the time the race starts, I am even with the lead runners. The end comes quickly, not ten yards into the race. I step in a drainage shaft hidden beneath a pile of leaves and severely twist my ankle. I try to ignore it, pretend it didn't happen. I continue to run.

By mile ten, my ankle seems swollen to the size of a small melon, and I am no longer able to put any weight on it at all. I finally succumb to the reality of what is happening and stop. I find an open spot on the curb and sit down. I am overwhelmed, beside myself. I do not know what to do. My mind is racing with thoughts about how I blew it, I am a failure, all the time I put in and the things I sacrificed all for nothing! How can I go home and face my friends, coworkers, and family?

On the brink of devastation and despair, I look up and watch the other runners flowing by, one after another. How I want to join them, be part of the event. I am at the point now that I don't even care about not running a great time. I just want to get back in and be part of the event.

I begin to fantasize on what I am doing in the race, what I hope to get out of it. Thoughts start flying through my mind, spontaneous and varied. I am transported away from the immediacy of the event to time immemorial. I am engaged in battle, marching with troops in a faraway place in a long ago time. I can either figure a way to go on or be left behind to the whims of fate.

Suddenly, I am back, sitting on the curb, staring at an aid station. What catches my eye are the buckets of ice that are being given to the runners to help cool them off. An idea begins to emerge. What if this race isn't about seeing how fast I can run? What if this event, and the things that happen to me while I am participating in it, are just a series of tests? And what if I conceive of these challenges as affording me the opportunity to delve into everything I know, use every resource I have to make the best out of every trial and tribulation that comes my way? What if, instead of feeling sorry for myself and dropping out of the race, I create another option for myself?

I make my way over to the aid station and ice down my ankle. After a few minutes the swelling in my ankle subsides, and I am feeling a little better. I begin to gingerly place some body weight on my ankle. I seem able to move a bit, so I start walking. Before I leave the aid station, I fill my sock with ice. To keep the ice in my sock, I tie my bandanna around the top. After a while, I am able to move, even run a bit.

All around me people are busy with their own races. Some runners turn to me and offer words of encouragement. Others tell me I am a fool for continuing to run on what—with all the ice packed in my sock—looks like a soccer ball growing out of my foot. I, too, am concerned about whether my decision to go on is going to damage my ankle. I monitor every step, making sure that I am not running through pain, but adjusting my pace, my foot placement, my distribution of body to keep the pain and discomfort at a minimum. I promise myself that if I start thinking I might be doing irreparable harm to my body I will stop. I want to run forever, not just for now. But I am confident that I can manage this moment and continue on, and I do.

I finish the race in four hours and three minutes. I am extraordinarily happy, probably more so than if I had simply run a great time. I guess part of me is much more curious about how I would handle unexpected adversity than how fast I could run 26.2 miles.

My journey doesn't end at the finish line. The process of living is an adventure that never ends, it incessantly and unrelentingly moves on. I ran today, and now I must ensure I can run tomorrow. I go back to my room and draw upon every bit of knowledge I can muster, every learned wisdom, every insightful experience and develop a life-affirming healing strategy. I soak my leg in ice for short periods of time and follow that with some yoga stretches and breathing exercises. After a few hours of this, I start a pattern of short warm baths, followed by equally short cool ones. I knew this would create a bellows effect in the circulatory and lymph system in my ankle and promote the removal of toxins and reduction in the swelling. By morning, the ankle is remarkably sound. I am able to jog a few miles, and I'm ready to move on to the next episode.

I am certain that everything that happens is for the better; everything that happens is for the good.

The message here isn't that you must finish the race at all costs, your health and well being be damned! Quite the contrary, what I got out of it—and the lesson I'd like to impart—is that in adversity there are possibilities, some of which we tend to overlook more easily than others. Keep your chin up and believe in yourself. Accept the challenge presented by the vicissitudes of life and you will always move forward, no matter what.

9

Follow the 85-Percent Rule

Of course you want to live life to the fullest and get the most out of every day. In the process, though, you must acknowledge that you cannot control it all. Be kind to yourself, and allow for the natural give-and-take of life. Accept the possibility that because of circumstances beyond your control, not everything you set out to do will go as planned. Part of life remains illusive, unpredictable, and unknowable.

This is especially true when it comes to your body—how you treat it and what you feed it. While it is admirable to want always to adhere to a particular program, it's neither necessary nor desirable. Excessive rigidity in your nutritional and training strategies can cost you the opportunity to discover something about yourself, make a new distinction, or benefit from an unexpected insight. If you define success in terms of adhering to the all-or-nothing rule of life, chances are you will lose motivation and excitement. Following your chosen plan can become tedious and dull. Instead of pursuing health and happiness, you can create heightened anxiety and stress that ultimately undermines the very reasons you set out on the voyage of health and vitality in the first place.

Certainly there are times when rigidity is necessary. If, for whatever reason, you have reached a point where your body is so out of balance that your health and well-being are threatened, by all means be resolute in your adherence to the plan. Sometimes, on your life's voyage, you may encounter severe turbulence and get thrown off course. In this state of imbalance, it doesn't take much adversity—consecutive missed running days, a week-long binge of toxic foods, an insidiously negative attitude—to completely confuse your direction. To get back on course, you must diligently and methodically get back to following your map. After, with a renewed sense of direction, you can retain your buoyancy and withstand the whims and vagaries of fate.

Create a plan that guides you to your goal yet is flexible enough to allow you to occasionally kick back. Be consistent in your commitment to your goals, and accept that every once in a while it is okay to step outside the context of your commitment and do something outrageous or even out of character. I would be lying to you if I told you I never did. Even in my most intensely competitive and productivity-driven stages, I allowed room for playfulness and acquiescence to social protocol that was not solely directed at achieving the prize. There has already been, and shall always be, the occasional shortened training session, a piece of birthday cake, a hot dog with my son Beau at a baseball game. To me, that's the meaning of the 85-percent rule.

It's late afternoon on a Saturday, and I'm in my office sitting by the computer in my workout clothes. I was going to run around noon, but I unexpectedly had to watch my little girl Mackenzie, who is playing in the other room. My wife was just called out of town for a last-minute business meeting, and I am taking over with the kids so she can take care of business. I was able to set my son up with a play date, but on such short notice, I couldn't do the same for my little girl. So she is with me, and I can't just disappear for the next two hours and go out for my daily afternoon run. Oh well, looks like I won't be able to get my run in today. What can I do? I can get all upset and cranky and complain to anyone and everyone around me how unfair it all is. Or I can roll with it and make the best of it. I've run a few hundred thousand miles; it's not a big deal if I can't squeeze in another ten or twelve. I take a deep breath and enjoy the moment I am sharing with my five-year-old daughter. I know how happy she is to spend the day with her daddy.

If setting a plan in motion and sticking to the plan is so important, how do you know when to deviate from the plan? One way is to rely on the innate wisdom of your body and your common sense. It's one thing to be fanatical and quite another to be passionate and joyful. Keep asking yourself, "What is the point?" "What am I doing this for?" The most powerful model comes from young children before they are shaped, molded, and hardened by the lessons taught in most conventional sports settings. Even within the confines of a structured workout or coaching session, most five-to-seven-year-olds will still figure out a way to tickle their buddies while the coach is making a serious attempt to explain a new technique or defensive strategy. The coach may be focusing on skill development, and the kids certainly do want to learn, but they also want to have fun. Most kids at that age don't really seem to have the one-thing-leads-to-another mentality that we grown-ups possess. For kids practice is fun, a time to be with the guys or gals, not just a way to insure greater success during the game. They don't yet understand they are working out. To them they're just playing—the foundation of which is pure joy and expression. Make sure you have some fun, too. If it means straying from the initial plan, so be it . . . as long as at least 85 percent of the time, you are consistent with the commitments you have in your life.

PART TWO

How to TRAIN
for the Distance

I am about to share with you the secret for accessing energy whenever you want it: just move! No matter how lethargic you feel or how much you don't want to exercise, you can always make yourself feel better by moving. Movement creates energy; it doesn't take it away. If you want the energy to sustain yourself on your life's journey, you can generate it by incorporating movement into every day.

Movement unlocks our senses, makes us feel alive, and allows us to rejoice in the here and now. We are physical beings, and we need to move. Humans and our bipedal ancestors have been around for hundreds of thousands of years. Yet it has only been in the last eighty or so years, since arming for the hunt or toiling in the fields was replaced by sitting at a desk in the industrialized countries, that motion has not been the norm of the day. With this decrease in daily physical activity, our bodies have become understimulated. Like a computer that goes into sleep mode when it isn't being used, many people settle into a state of lethargy and interpret their lack of energy as a sign that their body needs to be shut off or rested when, in reality, it's crying out to be used.

In this section, I will outline a training program that can evolve into many different forms, some more intricate than others. If you are just starting out and have never allowed movement to become a part of your life, the only thing that matters is that you find an activity that you enjoy doing and get out there and do it! It doesn't have to be complicated. Walk, run, bike, or swim. Stay comfortable, keep moving, and you will prosper. If you run but are not already engaged in a training program, I'll share techniques to make movement more effortless and joyful, simple, and sublime. If you're an experienced marathoner, open for new distinctions upon which to reorganize your training program, you can find them here. My system can be as complex or as simple as you like. I have added specific strategies designed to safeguard your journey as well as to make it spirited and fulfilling. These considerations include which shoes to wear, techniques to breathe more effectively, and how to interpret the various messages your body sends you as you interact with the physical world.

All the strategies I present are outgrowths of my lifelong commitment to physical training. I present them to you in the hope that you can learn to enjoy moving even more. Being physical shouldn't be just another chore or obligation. It doesn't have to be thought of as a discomfort that must be endured in order to gain some benefit down the road. Movement can be joyous and fun. It has its origins in childhood play, after all! Movement, and the experience it brings, is itself the reward and the desired outcome; it is not simply a means to some other end.

I am at a seminar in Hawaii, and I meet a workshop leader who claims she hates to exercise. She is such an energetic, vibrant woman, yet she is unhappy about her body. She feels so pressured about her weight, especially in the context of a seminar where everyone seems to be making commitments to better eating habits and regular exercise. The music is starting to play when she confesses her disdain for exercise. This makes her cry. She continues to sob as the music gets louder and the beat gets stronger. All around us people are dancing and celebrating. The spirit is infectious. Soon Molly, my unhappy friend, begins to get into the rhythm. She starts swaying to the music, along with everyone else. And there we both are, dancing and moving to the music. I look at her smiling and happy face, her state totally transformed by the festive environment. I lean over and give her a big hug and whisper that she never has to "exercise" again. All she needs to do is to think of movement as dancing. She smiles back and understands. Movement doesn't have to hurt to be good.

The next day, as the seminar is about to break for the afternoon lunch period, there is Molly walking on the path along the ocean, moving with a gleeful rhythm and style all her own, obviously feeling better about herself and her body. This is a powerful first step to getting her to see that "just moving" can be transformational.

That, my friend, is my goal. I want to transform physical training from something that you do because you think you have to into something you love so much you can no longer live without. So let us "move" on, and I'll show you how.

10

Ask Your Body What It Wants

Imagine being able to ask your body which exercise regime, nutritional strategy, pair of shoes, or even which cosmetic cream it wants. In a sense, this option is available. The body is always providing the mind with information about what it wants, needs, and doesn't want. However, most of us are out of touch with our bodies or just plain confused by its signals. To paraphrase John Gray, "Our bodies are from Mars, and our minds are from Venus."

Learning to access my body's innate wisdom helped me to discover the best treatment (you'd be surprised) for an injured knee, dramatically change my diet, and identify and clear up emotional stresses that interfered with my ability to perform. Developing this skill isn't difficult, and once you learn basic principles, you can test your body to discover what it desires and open up the possibility of alternative sources of treatment.

We routinely make decisions based on clues from the body. A classic clue is your stomach feeling as though it's ready to explode. Your body is sending a pretty clear message: "You've eaten enough!" So you stop eating. Or I bet you have noticed connections between what you eat and certain physical outcomes. For instance, every time my mom eats red meat, she has trouble sleeping. My wife gets the hiccups when she eats foods that are really spicy. A bowl of pasta or couple of slices of bread used to leave me bloated and sleepy. What about you? Have you observed connections between what you eat and negative physical outcomes? In these instances the body message is, "Don't eat those foods." To avoid the unpleasant symptoms, we avoid the foods.

Other signals, such as cravings, can be more ambiguous. Some experts maintain we crave the nutrients we need while others suggest cravings are based on an allergic reaction, meaning we crave foods to which we are allergic. To further complicate matters, we can crave a food because of a psychological dynamic. If your dad was a broccoli farmer and you heard the words "Eat your broccoli," at every meal, you may grow to detest broccoli. Or the opposite may be true. You might crave chocolate because it represents something your mom never let you eat when you were a child and now you're the one making the decisions.

The body gives equally ambiguous signals regarding exercise. Have you ever experienced an overwhelming fatigue at the end of a busy day? You interpret it as a sign that your body needs rest, so you skip the gym or walk and instead turn on the tube and give your body the evening off. But maybe that sluggishness is your body telling you that it needs to move more, not less.

And what is the body trying to tell us when we experience headaches, muscle aches, joint stiffness, allergies, flu symptoms, or digestive distress? Often, instead of finding out, we learn to live with the ailments and do our best to cover them up with drugs. We adjust our lifestyle to avoid the stress of movement and set ourselves up for further pain and immobility. Yet in the end, these chronic ailments deplete our energy and dampen our enthusiasm for being physical.

Applied kinesiology (AK), a diagnostic and treatment method developed by Dr. George Goodheart in the mid-1960s, is one pathway to better understanding our ever-present body signals. It uses muscle testing to balance the body and uncover internal ailments. AK presumes there are relationships between certain organs and certain muscles. The information a stiff muscle offers may well be more than just a gentle (maybe not so gentle) reminder that the next time you'd better be more prepared before working out. A weakness in your legs might be related to what you just ate and the stress it caused to your digestive system, not the fact you need to do more leg squats. Fatigue might be linked to a stressed-out organ, perhaps your liver or gall bladder.

Take knee pain, the number-one gripe among runners. Ask people who aren't runners what they think about when they hear the word *running*, and the first thing that pops into their head is knee pain. Running = knee pain. Most people interpret knee pain as a three-bell alarm screaming, "Don't run! Running isn't good for you! It damages your knees!"

If you consider that knee pain may mean something other than that the knee is damaged, you extend your options beyond suppressing the discomfort with pain killers, securing the joint with a knee brace, ceasing the activity until the pain goes away, or taking up another sport. Had I not had a life-changing episode involving knee pain, instead of pursuing a career as an ultradistance runner, I might have ended up sitting on a barstool, waxing poetic about my constant companion, Mister Pain-in-the-Knee.

It is January 1981, and I am running in New York City's Central Park with David Obelkovich, a fellow ultramarathoner who placed fifth in the national hundred-mile championships two years earlier. Out of nowhere, I begin to experience debilitating pain in my left knee. I cannot run even one more step. The pain is from the same knee that was injured and operated on after a skiing accident in 1975. The tip of my ski got stuck in the fresh, wet snow and the binding didn't release. I spun around on my left knee, with the ski ending up dangling somewhere above my right ear. I knew the moment it happened that I'd torn the ligaments in my knee. I had surgery to repair the ligaments and remove the cartilage. This was in the pre-arthroscopic surgery days, so the hospital stay lasted two weeks. Rehab started almost as soon as the anesthesia wore off and it took nearly five months before I could run again.

Now, almost exactly six years to the day of the accident, I experience an incapacitating, piercing pain in that same knee. David, an accomplished ultra-athlete, has the same fear as I, that this is the inevitable, career-ending injury— the logical outcome of constant wear and tear piled on top of a structurally weakened knee. David warns me, "Better go get that checked out." I thank him and take a cab home.

I rest, take aspirin, exercise on a stationary bike instead of run, get a massage a couple of times a week, include some extra weight training and stretching and hope that my knee gets better. It doesn't though. I am miserable. Nothing I do replaces the euphoria I get when I run. Days turn into weeks, and weeks turn into months. I still can't run.

Hoping for a miracle cure, I see the surgeon who per-formed the knee surgery. After examining an x-ray, he reminds me, "You have no cartilage." He continues, "The wear and tear has begun to leave deposits in your knee, mak-ing it resemble the arthritic knee of a much older man." He emphasizes his point by waving his fingers underneath the markings on the x-ray to indicate where the deposits are beginning to form in my knee joint. He warns me that I will be crippled by age forty if I continue to run such long dis-tances.

I am twenty-nine years old at the time, already running more than a hundred miles a week.

By March, I am willing to try almost anything. My friend Brian Flanagan recommends that I see a chiroprac-tor. I end up going to a chiropractic physician, Avery

Ferentz, who was trained in applied kinesiology. Through Avery, I become exposed to this holistic and integrated approach of understanding what might be happening in my body. I begin to recognize that a painful joint or a weak and tired muscle might have prior causes that I had not even thought about. Lifestyle factors such as what I eat and how I deal with stress—indeed how healthy I am—affect how well my knee feels. Certainly the pain in my knee was real and tangible. But I was now being led to believe that factors besides running and the damage caused by the skiing accident were involved. The factors had to do with my health as opposed to my fitness, a distinction made to me by Phil Maffetone.

Understanding the difference between health and fitness is critical. Fitness is a relative measure of physical performance compared to some form of standard. Fitness is assessed in terms of such measures as how many push-ups or sit-ups you can do, how strong your legs are, or how fast you can run a mile. Health is different. Health has to do with how well the various systems of the body function. These systems include the following:

- **Digestive**—how successfully you absorb the nutrients you eat
- **Immune**—how well you are able to ward off illness and disease
- **Lymph**—how effectively your body carries away the toxins produced as your body tries to protect itself from damage by foreign materials
- **Adrenal**—how reliably your body is able to manage and cope with stress
- **Nervous**—how dependably your brain and nervous system communicate with the rest of your body
- **Musculoskeletal**—how reasonably your muscles and bones function, allowing you to move and distribute energy

as your body supports itself against gravity and participates in the physical world

It is possible for a person to be fit—able to run fast, lift an extraordinary amount of weight, and have big, bulging muscles—and not be healthy. For example, if your liver is stressed, your immune system weak, and your adrenal glands exhausted, no matter how fit you are—no matter how many push-ups you can do, or sit-ups you can perform—your quality of life gets diminished. Your energy and vitality will waver, your body will ache, and you'll function far below optimal efficiency. Avery challenged me to accept that the way my body felt might be a reflection of what went on inside.

The distinction between health and fitness led me to a different way of understanding typical symptoms of pain and discomfort. Pain and discomfort are windows of opportunity through which we can gain insight into the internal workings of the body. Everything in the body is related; everything is one.

A symptom of structural imbalance, say knee pain, can derive from a dysfunctional internal organ exacerbated by poor nutrition and emotional distress. The reverse is also true. Mood state can influence the health of our internal organs, which can manifest itself in joint pain. For example, chronic stress can lead to adrenal exhaustion and medial (inside) knee discomfort.

I start to recognize that I am out of whack. My entire being is wrapped up in my identity as a successful runner. Not only do I strive to win at all times, I *must* win in order to feel significant. I am driven. To regain my health, I need to relax, enjoy being a runner, instead of needing to be a winner. My diet, though disciplined to some extent, stinks. I live on the typical runner's diet of pasta, bread, potatoes, beer, coffee, and a pint of Häagen Dazs every night. Not only do I exercise intensely, but also for what could be considered insanely long periods of time. The combination of emotional stress of needing to succeed, nutritional imbalance, and excessive physical activity creates enormous strain on my internal organs. In this case, my adrenal glands are most affected.

Stress and Your Adrenal Glands

Before I go further, I must explain what the adrenal glands are and what purpose they serve in the body. Once you understand how the adrenals affect the way your body feels, what to do about it will be clear.

The adrenal glands, located above each kidney, are flattened, cap-like tissues that help to manage stress by secreting hormones that stabilize the blood-sugar level. These hormones affect the heart, blood vessels, other glands, and nervous system. Some of these hormones are called catecholemines, composed of norepinephrine (NE) and epinephrine (E), which serve to either excite (E) or calm down (NE) the nervous system. Other hormones, mineralocorticoids (specifically corticosterone) serve as antiinflammatory agents that can alleviate the amount of pain and discomfort associated with physical training.

The adrenals also secrete a hormone that stabilizes blood sugar during periods of stress. This hormone (a glucocorticoid) is called cortisol, which is a glucose synthesizer and stimulates the production of more blood sugar. Under normally functioning conditions, cortisol also prevents existing blood sugar from being used up and encourages the body to burn fat instead. It raises the level of protein carried by the blood in order to promote tissue repair and growth.

However, cortisol does have a significant downside once levels get high or the adrenals are asked to perform their stress-management functions too often. Cortisol is an inflammatory agent that inhibits circulation and is an immune-system suppressant.

When stress is constant and excessive, the adrenal glands don't function well. Stress can come from a wide variety of sources—emotional, physiological, and nutritional. Refer to the box that follows for a list of factors that can cause adrenal strain and dysfunction.

FACTORS LEADING TO ADRENAL STRESS

Constant flight-or-fight stress
Emotional problems (familial, social, financial)
Problems at work
Work overload
Relationship problems
A diet high in caffeine, sugar, white flour, soft drinks
Excessive anaerobic exercise; repetitive bouts of sugar-
burning exercise

Hans Selye's Three Stages of Adrenal Stress Reaction

Hans Selye is a Canadian scientist best known for his research on how the human body copes with and manages stress. He developed a theory related to the way the adrenals react to stress. The first stage of this reaction is called the alarm reaction. At the onset of stress, the adrenals are summoned to secrete hormones and stabilize blood sugar levels, thus reducing pain and discomfort. However, if the stress is chronic or increases and the adrenals cannot secrete enough hormones to cope with the stress, the adrenals enter the second stage of adaptation, called the resistance stage.

During the resistance stage, the adrenals actually enlarge—a process called hypertrophy—like a muscle does during periods of constant and repetitive stimulation. At this point, the adrenals have been fighting a losing battle, so the body enlarges the whole gland just to keep up with the stress. The final stage of the adrenal glands' adaptation to stress is exhaustion. The battle is lost. The white flag goes up. The adrenal glands can no longer adapt to stress. Symptoms now appear chronic: mental and physical fatigue set in; joint pain intensifies (particularly the knee, lower back, and foot); and allergies, colds, and flu-like symptoms linger. As the adrenals experience "burnout," the sartorius muscle weakens. The sartorius wraps around the upper thigh and connects the outside of the hip to the inside of the knee. If the sartorius weakens, the knee becomes unstable, and knee pain results. The pain is most noticeable on the inside (medial) portion of the knee where the sartorius inserts. The phenomenon of "knees knocking" under duress is an example of the sartorius muscle weakening.

My dysfunctional adrenals had begun to adversely affect me by weakening the sartorius muscle. As the sartorius weakened, my knee became unstable, and knee pain developed precisely where medial collateral ligament was surgically repaired. I was tempted to conclude the obvious, that the pain in my knee was no more than the outcome of a skiing accident and subsequent surgery. However, the equation of "skiing accident + surgery = no running" was not an acceptable outcome to me. I embraced therapies that acknowledge that a combination of nutritional, emotional, and lifestyle-related stressors might be affecting the muscles that stabilize the knee, putting me at risk and, ultimately, in pain.

My doctor used muscle testing to find out which organs and glands might be stressed out and therefore affecting the workings of the muscles and bones. He stimulated accupressure points to release stress inside my body, strengthen my muscles, and stabilize my knee. Both Max and Avery were certain that the portents of doom cast upon me by the orthopedic surgeon must not be accepted as gospel. They encouraged a combination of positive thinking, improved eating habits, nutritional supplements, and other adjustments to promote optimal organ function and energy flow throughout my body.

Please understand me: I am not proposing that all knee pain can be alleviated through chiropractic, muscle testing, balanced nutrition, managing stress better, and positive thinking. Nor did I conclude that at the time. I was amazed, though, that knee discomfort so debilitating and painful one minute could disappear as if by magic the next. Something remarkable did happen.

A week after these therapies, I was back up to twenty miles a day. By June, six months after the setback in Central Park, I was running more than thirty miles a day and broke my own American hundred-mile road racing record by four minutes (a hundred miles in thirteen hours and four seconds). Two years later, I entered my first multiday race and started running really long distances—all on a surgically repaired knee, with the cartilage removed! I owe it all to the health-care professionals who introduced me to the possibility that the conventional wisdom might not be as empowering as the unconventional. Indeed, by using muscle testing to access the innate wisdom of my own body, I was able to go on to a career that would not have been possible had I relied solely on conventional medical science.

Perhaps the common knee discomfort experienced by so many runners—indeed, athletes of all kinds—is related to something other than the running motion or "pounding" on the ground, as is so commonly thought. Whenever I meet people who say, "Every time I start running, I get knee pain, so I don't run anymore," I consider it a tragedy. I absolutely believe we are "born to run." To me, removing such a fundamental and basic human act from the options we have in life arbitrarily reduces the possibilities we have for joy and fulfillment. For the moment, though, all I ask is for you to consider is a simple proposition: perhaps the prevalence of knee pain is not due to the inevitability of the "running = knee pain" formula. Perhaps other factors may be involved.

Modern Western society is the most stressful in history. Stress is so common it could be considered an indelible aspect of the culture. Too many people work too many hours, eat excessive amounts of sugar, don't get enough quality rest, breathe in polluted air, or consume foods containing pesticides, preservatives, and other questionable chemicals. Is it such a stretch to conclude that the scope of adrenal disfunction and digestive distress might be nearly epidemic? Under these conditions, when a person undertakes a physically demanding task, a muscle, already weakened by internal or external stress, can break down. Conventional medicine might look at a case of chronic knee pain and not find anything wrong with the knee joint itself, leaving no viable treatment options other than pain killers, braces, or restricting movement. There is another option, though. Once it is established that the knee pain is not being treated successfully with conventional methodologies—and there is no noticeable trauma or structural damage—you might, as I did, consider consulting with an alternative health practitioner, especially one who is certified in applied kinesiology, who can explore the inherent wisdom of the body with you.

The Science of Muscle Testing

Muscle testing as a means to access information about the body is largely based on the work of Dr. George Goodheart. Goodheart is generally accredited with establishing the discipline of applied kinesiology (AK). Every time I say that name, I am amazed at how the universe works—that such a wonderful human being could have such an appropriate name, Goodheart.

Goodheart promoted the use of muscle testing as a diagnostic and treatment tool for physicians and other health-care providers. He bases his AK techniques on an observed relationship between specific muscle groups and internal organ systems. By first isolating a muscle and then manually applying gradually increasing pressure against a muscle, Goodheart evaluates the strength and weakness of a particular muscle. A strong muscle means that the associated organ is functioning well, a weak muscle that the organ is not. Thus, Goodheart believes we can gain access to what is going on in the body. As mentioned earlier, Goodheart believes that each specific muscle is linked to a specific organ via a shared nervous system web and network of blood vessels. Information flow between organ and muscle is incessant and instantaneous. He accepts the notion that the health of muscle is determined by the health of the organ. By testing the relative degree of muscle strength and weakness, the muscle tester is able to diagnose the relative health and function of the internal organ and vice versa.

Now I must point out that there exists a whole world of medical practitioners who don't believe the health of an internal organ can affect the strength of a specific muscle. I remember quite vividly what my internist said when I questioned him about the correlation: "Preposterous." Before my knee trauma I, too, shared his reaction. Clearly, my position on this has changed dramatically over the years.

Goodheart and his followers have uncovered a number of significant organ-to-muscle relationships. The health and function of the following organs are linked to the strength and weakness of a specific associated muscle. The chart below identifies some of the most important associations between various organs and glands and the muscle groups to which they are related.

Organ/Glandular System	Muscle Affected	Typical Complaint When Organ Is Dysfunctional
Adrenal	Sartorius	Medial knee pain (on inside of knee)
Gall Bladder	Popliteus	Pain in back of knee
Large Intestine/Colon	Hamstrings	Back problems, lower body fatigue
Small Intestine	Quadriceps	Back problems, lower body fatigue
Bladder	Tibialis Anterior	Ankle instability, back problems
Sex Organs	Gluteus Maximus	Lower back problems, lack of muscle tone in the abdomen
Sex Organs	Piriformis	Pain up and down the sciatic nerve web
Liver	Pectoralis Major (Chest)	Headaches, fatigue
Liver	Rhomboids (Shoulderblades)	Upper back strain
Kidney	Psoas	Lower back pain

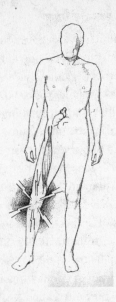

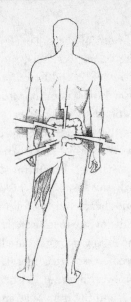

Knee pain can be caused by stressed-out adrenal glands, which weaken the sartorius muscle. (The sartorius originates at the hip, wraps around the thigh, and inserts into the inside of the knee.)

Colon irritation can weaken the hamstrings and cause back pain.

The Digestive System and Large Muscles of the Lower Body

Ask any runner who gets diarrhea or digestive problems how his legs feel, and I venture to say the answer is "less than at peak level." That's because the health of the digestive system governs the strength of the large muscles of the lower body, including the hamstring (back of the upper leg) and quadriceps (thigh) muscle. Early in my running career, I learned to eat in ways that promoted digestive health. I still avoid acid-forming foods such as most fruits and concentrated fruit juices, fried foods, fatty meats, candy bars, and caffeine. As long as my stomach is healthy, so are my legs. If my legs are healthy, my energy never leaves.

It's important to note that while a dysfunctional organ will influence the health of its related muscle group, the reverse is not always true. For instance, if you're on a downhill trail run, the excessive stress experienced by the quadriceps can cause muscular discomfort but not necessarily digestive distress. However, if you attempt to complete a task that requires you to be on your feet for a long time, make sure you treat your digestive tract well before you set out on your journey.

In 1998 I had the pleasure to meet Dr. Goodheart while I was participating in a research project funded by his organization the International College of Applied Kinesiology (ICAK). As the data gathering was drawing to a close, I was introduced to him by one of my colleagues. I had been waiting years for this moment, having been aware of Goodheart's work for nearly fifteen years.

"I have to ask you this one question," I said to Goodheart, who nodded back to me. He had an amazing presence, strong hands, and a marvelous energy that was both focused and calm. "It's the 'Ah-Hah!' question I am curious about. Do you remember the moment when the relationship between the muscles and the internal organs became apparent to you and you went 'Ah-Hah! I got it!'?"

He answered by telling me this story: early in his career as a chiropractor, he had a cluster of patients with similar thyroid dysfunction, and they all displayed a similar posture. He then let his arms hang by his side, and, turning his hands outward, began mimicking the pose that a typical thyroid patient would strike. He then went on to notice a similar phenomenon occurring with a few of his patients, who all had the same kidney ailment. They, too, began to adopt a similar posture, albeit a different one from the thyroid patients.

These observations led Goodheart to conclude that dysfunction in certain organs influence the way the muscles work. He then theorized that he could improve the function of the organ by treating the muscle. Goodheart was able to make the jump from his observations of patient postures and organ disease to the development of a new and innovative treatment modality because of his understanding of human physiology. Already convinced that the health of muscles is inextricably linked to the health of the organs, Goodheart hypothesized that he could affect the function of an organ by working on the muscle.

Certainly there are challenges to using muscle testing: the tester may be biased or the person being tested may or may not be open to the treatment or may eventually experience fatigue from the process. However, these same criticisms could be brought to bear on the conventional doctor-patient relationship. There seems to me to be a sobering similarity between the deceitful alternative health-care practitioner who utilizes muscle-testing technologies and the preoccupied physician who routinely subscribes to a wide variety of conventional diagnostic testing. Certainly, muscle testing might have been used in the past to promote the sale of supplements and products that are not really needed. However, the same criticism can be leveled against a conventional medical approach that often routinely promotes prescription-drug therapies and surgery to vanquish symptoms that might be better off dealt with by lifestyle changes such as exercise, stress management, and better food choice. The diagnostic tools of both the conventional and alternative variety can be used either constructively or disingenuously. It is the responsibility of both the practitioner and the patient to ensure that the tools are used for good. The bottom line is that we must not lose out on the potential benefits of the enlightened application of a powerful new technology out of fear of its misuse.

Goodheart went on to form the International College of Applied Kinesiology (ICAK), which was primarily designed to educate and train physicians and health-care professionals. His work influenced others, including John Thie, D.C., who refined Goodheart's work under the rubric "Touch for Health." Touch for Health (TFH), based on the muscle-testing fundamentals of applied kinesiology (AK), extends muscle testing to include a system of accupressure point stimulation and simple massage techniques to relieve pain, enhance energy, and promote health. John

Maguire, the director of the Kinesiology Institute in San Diego, California, distinguishes the two different but related approaches this way: "Goodheart's system is for doctors; Thie's work is available and accessible to the layperson."

What makes these technologies so distinctive is their reliance on the use of muscle testing to get information about what is going on in the fundamental areas of organ function, structure balance (muscles and bones), nutrition, energy, and emotion. Muscle testing is used to direct the most appropriate treatment therapies, nutritional strategies, training regimens, and mindset practices. All this is accomplished by using a safe, noninvasive, holistic methodology that treats the muscles as a biofeedback meter to the inner sanctums of the body.

I am aware that the scope with which many practitioners (and I) have used muscle testing has gone far beyond what was originally conceived and intended by Goodheart and his organization. Testing a muscle to get information about the health and function of an organ is one thing. Testing a muscle to get information about whether a person should eat bananas instead of oranges might be quite another. Yet the body's innate intelligence is always operative, and the logic behind such an assertion may not be as far-fetched as you might think.

Since my first exposure to muscle testing technologies in the early 1980s, I have had the pleasure to have worked with (and be worked on by) many brilliant health professionals who use muscle-testing technologies in a wide variety of ways. Herbie Ross, D.C., an alternative-health physician based in Miami, once paid Goodheart for the privilege of following him around for a week as he performed his rounds. Ross explains the phenomenon of a muscle strengthening or weakening upon coming in touch with certain substance in terms of energy frequencies. Ross views the body as a spectrometer—a processor of energy frequencies emitted by all matter, animate or inanimate. He believes that once in contact with any substance, the body analyzes its frequency to determine its compatibility with that substance. The process is immediate and instantaneous.

Maguire teaches the process of entering a substance into your body's "circuitry"—a fancy word for its information-processing system. Once the substance is entered into the circuitry—and your body becomes aware of it—an instantaneous feedback loop between the conscious mind and the instinctive body is established. Maguire, too, is convinced that the body is always "talking" to us, offering clues as to whether a substance is "energizing" or "deenergizing." When a substance is energizing, your body will tell you by maintaining or increasing strength in the muscle being tested. When a substance is deenergizing, the muscle weakens.

A Los Angeles chiropractor who once worked on me and a number of my clients used to amaze me by recommending nutrients simply by noting the body language of the person holding the supplement in his or her hand. A slight change in the coloring of the face, a tensing of the muscles in the forehead, or the drooping of a shoulder were some of the changes he noticed. Depending on the particular reaction, he was able to gauge whether the body was accepting or rejecting a particular nutrient. "This one your body seems to like," he would declare. Or "I don't think your body wants that one." Using this methodology, he once diagnosed a close friend of mine with a prostate weakness, which was later verified by a urologist. Amazing! Again, all this is based on the principle in physics that all matter is energy. Your body will tell you if the energy of a substance is compatible with your system by either strengthening or weakening it. I knew firsthand, through my work with Avery and later with my good friend and colleague, Phil Maffetone, how powerful muscle-testing techniques could be. I came to rely on muscle testing as a tool to determine which supplements and treatment modalities worked best.

Throughout my multiday running career, Phil successfully used muscle-testing techniques on me to discover and redress imbalance and dysfunction in my body, to detect which foods to use, and to decide which shoes to wear. Based on the muscle "yes/no" response—a strengthened muscle meant the supplement worked, a weakened response meant it didn't—the practitioner could rely on the inherent wisdom of the body to direct the patient toward the proper treatment.

How to Ask Your Body What It Wants

It is not the intention of this book to teach applied kinesiology to diagnose organ dysfunction or to treat muscular skeletal pain and discomfort. AK is a complex system of diagnosis and treatment that takes years of study and practice to master. Professionals such as Maguire at the Kinesiology Institute or Goodheart's group at the International College of Applied Kinesiology (ICAK), can accommodate you or refer you to the proper training and certification programs.

However, I do believe that each and every one of us can master simple muscle-testing techniques that can more directly "tune" us into what our bodies are trying to say. The muscle tests I am going to describe below are more of the yes/no variety. Does your body like this nutrient, pair of shoes, or workout regime? If the muscle gets stronger or remains the same, yes. If the muscle weakens, no.

The responses you get from the muscle testing are not infallible, nor are they intended to override other information and advice. Each one of us must still actively participate in the decisions we make about what to do when it comes to feeding, treating, and physically challenging the body. There may be times when the results of a particular muscle test so radically contradict what we believe or what a trusted friend or conventional physician says that we might regard them with caution and even choose another path. That's okay. It doesn't mean that muscle testing or the friend or physician is wrong. It only means that you still have to choose what you think is best. I just prefer having some input from my body about what it wants before I make a decision.

The muscle-testing technique described below is not a strength test in the conventional sense. Do not approach testing of this nature with the mentality of an arm wrestler. Muscle testing does not seek to determine who is stronger, the tester or the person being tested. The question we are asking is clear and uncomplicated. Does coming into contact with a particular substance—whether it be a piece of food, nutritional supplement, pair of shoes, or energy-replacement fluid—affect the function of the muscle by strengthening or weakening it as a gradually increasing force is placed against it? You must first make sure that the person being tested has no injuries or physical challenges that might be adversely affected by a muscle-testing procedure. Make sure you ask the person being tested if he or she might be at risk if you test a particular muscle.

Once you have the go-ahead, you can gauge the correct amount of force to exert against a selected indicator muscle by keeping the pressure around two to four pounds. Here's a helpful benchmark: most adult arms weight between one and two pounds, so the feeling should be one to four times the amount of effort it takes to just hold your arm up, perpendicular to your body. Another neat trick is to either imagine or actually practice using a postal scale. Place your hand on the top of the scale, arm straight, hand extended. Starting very easily, gradually increase the pressure and push down on the top of the scale until you reach four pounds. Then ease up and go back down to one pound. Repeat. After three to five trials, you will be better at keeping the tension in the desired range.

The selection of the indicator muscle is next. Most often the shoulder muscle (deltoid) is selected. The delts are readily accessible and quite easy to use. The person being tested needs only to stand or sit comfortably and hold his or her arm out to the side, perpendicular to the body—or in front, angled down at approximately a forty-five-degree angle.

Keep the elbow locked, with the palms open and facing down. Once again, make sure that you ask if the person you are testing has a current or past history of shoulder discomfort. Only after it is established that there is little or no risk to the shoulder should you proceed.

Other muscles can be substituted if, for some reason, the deltoid muscle isn't appropriate. For instance, drop your arm down by your side, keep your elbow straight, and have your palm facing your body to isolate the large muscle of your upper back (the lats). Your partner can activate the upper back muscle by grasping your arm just above the wrist and trying to pull your arm away from your body.

The Muscle-Test Procedure

- Isolate an indicator muscle, most often the deltoid muscle.
- Have your subject extend arm to side, perpendicular to body or in front at a forty-five-degree angle, elbows locked, palm face down.
- Gradually apply increasing pressure (one to four pounds) just above the subject's wrist.
- As gradually increasing pressure is being applied, the subject exhales.
- If muscle is unblocked, the muscle will be able to resist the gradually increasing pressure; if the muscle is blocked, it will weaken and no longer be able to resist.

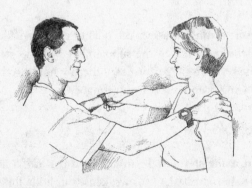

Calibrating the Yes/No Response

- Assume the test position described above. Have the person being tested stand or sit comfortably and hold his or her arm out to the side, perpendicular to the body. Keep the elbow locked, with the palms open and facing down.
- Have subject state his/her own name. My name is _____.
- Test muscle by gradually applying between two to four pounds of pressure. The muscle should be able to resist pressure.
- Have subject make up a fictitious name and claim that the made-up name is his/hers. My name is _____.
- Retest the muscle. The muscle should weaken and no longer be able to resist the gradually increasing pressure.

For best results, the subject must maintain a relaxed state of anticipation and detached curiosity about what the body is about to reveal. As stated at the outset of this chapter, muscle testing has widespread applications. By applying pressure to various pressure points, you can find out if a particular nutrient, piece of athletic equipment, or even sunscreen is compatible with your system. When it comes in contact with a substance, your body immediately gives you information whether it likes a substance.

Supplements:

Use muscle testing to assess the quality of a particular supplement or if the ingestion of the supplement will add stress to the system. The test can be performed either by holding the supplement or placing it underneath your tongue.

Shoe fit and model:

Try on running shoes, walk around, and perform a muscle test to see if the shoe strengthens or weakens your body function.

Sports equipment:

Hold a tennis racquet, golf club, or sit on a bike, and then test your muscles to see if the equipment promotes optimal body structure.

Cosmetics, lotions, sunscreens:

Put a dollop of a cream in your hand, and then test the muscle to ascertain the feedback from your body.

DOES A SPECIFIC FOOD ADD OR DRAIN ENERGY FROM THE BODY?

• Assume testing position. Enter the food into the "circuitry of the system" by holding the food (against the jaw, or over the thymus gland, about where the second button of a shirt would be), tasting, smelling, or even thinking of the food.
• Place the first two fingers of the tester's free hand around the back of the subject on the top of the neck, just off of the spine, under the base of the skull. (This asks the body if any system in the body will be stressed by the consumption of this particular food.)
• Follow the same muscle-testing technique outlined earlier.

Touch for Health as Preventive Medicine

Many athletes use touch-for-health practice as outlined by Dr. John Thei throughout the day to find where stress is stored in the body and then apply pressure to release it.

Maguire recommends stimulating specific accupressure or reflex points in order to promote energy release and the optimal functioning of the corresponding organs and muscles. These reflex points act as the body's energy terminals, directing the flow of energy through a network of energy pathways or meridians. Should the energy terminal get switched off, by, say, a distressed or dysfunctional organ, the energy flow gets blocked, and the associated muscles weakens. These switches can be turned back on and the energy flow unblocked by stimulating the reflex points with the application of gentle pressure by the fingers, usually in a tight circular motion with the thumb or index finger.

Reflex points for the key organ groups of adrenals, liver, kidney, colon, and stomach are located above and approximately one inch to the left and right of the navel. Closest to the navel and below the other two are the kidney pressure points (or reflexes). One inch above the kidney reflex points are the adrenal points (one inch to the left and right and two inches above the navel). Three inches above and one inch to the left and right of the navel are the reflex points for the liver. Stimulation of tender accupressure points for twenty to thirty seconds two to three times a day activates lymphatic (the body's sewage system), blood, and energy flow to the muscles, organs, and glands. For daily maintenance, stimulate all the reflexes identified in the following illustration for three to five seconds. If a spot is especially tender, continue to "work" the spot for sixty seconds or until the tenderness is reduced. During athletic competition, stimulation can continue for two to three minutes.

Maguire and Nate Zinsser, Ph.D., a noted sports psychologist and director of the Center for Enhanced Performance at the United States Military Academy, recommend that you periodically inventory the body for tender spots along the noted reflex point meridians. Nate has been and continues to be actively involved in my running career as a trusted confidant, friend, and member of my racing crew. "If a spot is sore, go to it," Nate always says. I am sure he is influenced as much by his formal academic training as he is by more than thirty years of practicing and teaching Shotokan karate and his extraordinary career as an adventurer and mountain climber.

REFLEX POINTS

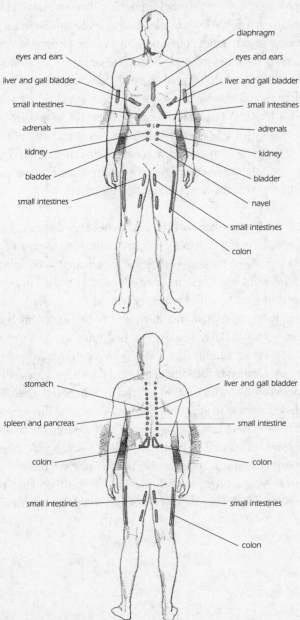

diaphragm

eyes and ears

eyes and ears

liver and gall bladder

liver and gall bladder

small intestines

small intestines

adrenals

adrenals

kidney

kidney

bladder

bladder

navel

small intestines

small intestines

colon

stomach

liver and gall bladder

spleen and pancreas

small intestine

colon

colon

small intestines

small intestines

colon

John Maguire is the same way. He preaches allocating time on a regular basis to relate to the body tactilely and tangibly. By discovering and self-treating blocked reflex points, one can promote optimal health and maintain superior energy. Simple massage techniques such as "feathering" (lightly brushing the affected area with one's fingertips) are used to alleviate stress and tension, release muscle cramps, and reduce pain.

Throughout this book I'll refer to muscle testing as a means of testing what your body really wants and to detect the potential causes of nagging ailments—and treat them accordingly. Muscle-testing technologies have saved me more than once in my career, and I'd like to share with you the following story.

It is the last few hours of the La Rochelle six-day race. I am in the lead, certain to win for the first time. For the past three days I have been battling with a severe pain that runs up and down my right leg. Then my knee goes out. I think, "I'm going to win, but I can't walk!" I remember the adrenal pressure point located in my abdomen, just above and to the left of my belly button, which an AK practitioner had once used on me to release some discomfort that had appeared in a similar spot on my knee. Desperate for some relief, and driven by a passionate desire to complete this most wonderful moment on my two feet running, I recruit an athletic trainer from the local French soccer team and have him massage the point. I am sure the trainer, who speaks no English, is at first a little taken aback by my incessant pointing at my stomach, but soon he catches on and begins massaging the area I show him. Within moments, the knee is stabilized. I am back in shape and win the race with 536 miles.

11

Always Buy a Shoe Fit, Not a Shoe Size

I can spend hours and hours with clients, discussing every facet of their mindset, training, and diet, and what's often the most important distinction they take away? They have been in the wrong shoes. Believe me, I do not consider that a minimal outcome. Choosing a pair of shoes that fit can mean the difference between comfort and injury. I have seen too many people organize an ambitious training regimen and follow a well-balanced nutritional program only to break down because their shoes don't fit. I know this firsthand because it happened to me.

During the Rocky Mountain six-day race, which began on December 27, 1984, and ended on January 2, 1985, I made my first serious attempt at running a hundred miles a day for six straight days. I almost made it! I had 504 miles going into day six, making my goal well within reach. But I broke down. My Achilles tendon, the area between my heel and lower calf muscle, became extremely painful. I had difficulty supporting my body weight on my right side. Even with Phil Maffetone's magic bodywork, I could not alleviate the pain. In the end, I managed to cover "only" 73.75 miles on the final day. Still, I finished with 577.75 miles, which remains the modern-day American record.

After the race, Phil and I reviewed the strategy. We were joined by a fascinating man named Dick Schwartz, a pedorthist from New Jersey who designs orthopedic shoes and foot-care products for his company, Apex Foot Health Industries. (A pedorthist is trained in foot anatomy and the construction of shoes and foot orthotic devices.) Dick considered long-distance endurance challenges the ultimate testing ground for foot-care products, much in the same way that the Indy 500 is used as a testing-ground (and marketing tool) for automobile products. Dick examined my shoes and feet and concluded my Achilles tendon pain was the result of shoes that were too small. I was racing (at age thirty-three then) in a size ten and-a-half shoe, a size I had been wearing since I stopped growing in high school. We had not given much thought to changing a shoe size that had seemingly worked all these years. With some simple tests, we discovered I would be better served by increasing my shoe size to a twelve. Yes, nearly two full sizes!

You see, in order to promote optimal muscular and skeletal health and function, the body needs to direct the muscular skeletal stress caused by holding itself up against the force of gravity down the spine and out the feet. The biomechanics of the foot play a crucial role in determining how well the body dissipates this stress. The foot needs to slide forward and the toes need to spread out as your body weight propels you forward. Enough room is required in the toe box in order to perform this function. If the shoe is too short or narrow, the toes get "jammed" and the forward and outward energy flow is disrupted. Instead of moving energy and stress down, through, and out the body, this "toe jamming" ricochets the energy off the front of the shoe and back up the skeletal system. Shoes that are too small and narrow do not encourage optimal biomechanical function of the foot, disrupting the natural energy flow of the body and potentially causing injury and discomfort.

How did I, someone who spent hours and hours dissecting each and every aspect of my running, get stuck in shoes that were too short? Easily, just like most of the people I have come in contact with over the years. Maffetone calls it the short-shoe syndrome. Most of us are influenced by it. In our culture, most people have the same attitude about their shoes as they do about their weight or their waistline—smaller is better. So as members of the short-shoe-syndrome culture, we choose smaller instead of larger size shoes. We all want to believe we have smaller, daintier feet, as if large feet were somehow less appealing and smaller feet sexier.

Over the years my wife, Mary Beth, and I have performed thousands of foot evaluations and found the vast majority of people wear shoes that are way too small. To determine the right shoe size, most often we use a device called a foot imprinter. The imprinter has a rubber pad that is inked from below. Blank paper is placed under the inked pad and the person whose feet are being analyzed simply walks over the pad. The pressure from the foot then leaves an ink impression on the paper. We use this information for shoe fitting as well as to assess the weight bearing and biomechanical patterns of the foot. Later, I will describe a simple way to perform a similar test at home.

When we suggest that a person increase his or her shoe length, often by as much as one to two full sizes, almost always we later get a call with the comment, "I can't believe I once jammed my feet into a space that small." I absolutely believe there is a version of Murphy's Law operative here: "Your feet will expand to fill the space available to them."

During my seminars or in private sessions, I often draw attention to my size-twelve shoes, quite noticeable on my five-foot-nine-inch frame. I have the shoes tied-up snugly, but not tight—loose enough to literally slide in-and-out of, like a pair of loafers. I tied my shoes too tightly during an event, and as my foot swelled from being on my feet for hours, I managed to impair circulation, which caused a whole bunch of problems. I will never do that again. I highly recommend not tying your shoelaces too tightly. I see this a lot. People try to tie their laces as tightly as possible, as if the extra firmness will stabilize the foot better. In most cases, the natural structure of your feet and ankles will stabilize your body. Think of your exercise shoes as fitting more like a slipper than a glove. While I do not recommend such a slipper-like feel for sports that demand constant side-to-side movement, such as tennis, soccer, basketball, baseball, and football, I do encourage it for straight-ahead activities like walking and running.

Another explanation of short-shoe syndrome stems from our tendency to buy a shoe size that we have been wearing for years rather than consciously participating in a decision to select a shoe based on comfort. The truth is that as you get healthier and fitter, your feet get bigger. The healthier, fitter body is in greater balance. Body weight is more evenly distributed, and the feet tend to spread out over a greater surface area. Understanding this is critical. It is important to remember this phrase: "Always by a fit, not a size."

Not only can the health and fitness of a person affect the size and shape of the foot, so can factors such as dehydration, stress, and the amount of time spent on the feet. Toward the latter stages of my multiday racing career, I usually brought along a range of running-shoe sizes to the event, in half-size increments, from twelve to thirteen. Usually, as the event progressed, I would increase the size of my shoe to accommodate changes in the size of my foot. I used to joke to my handlers that if I kept running, my feet would eventually be longer than my height.

How to Choose the Right Shoe

STEP 1

Always shop for shoes toward the end of the day, when your foot may be slightly bigger rather than earlier, when your foot is smaller. Err on the side of the shoe being a little bit too large rather than too small. With this in mind, if one foot is larger than the other (which is usually the case—few people evenly distribute their body weight left-to-right side) fit the pair of shoes to the larger foot.

STEP 2

If possible, get your feet measured with a Brannock device. You might remember the Brannock device from when you were a kid. It is usually a silver metal apparatus that measures the length and width of a shoe. Most conventional measuring devices calculate the length of the foot, or what is technically called the heel-to-toe distance. The Brannock device also provides the heel-to-ball measurement, which is quite important. It measures where the widest part of your foot (the ball) is in relationship to the length of the shoe (heel-to-toe). For instance, if your foot measures a size eleven heel-to-ball, the widest part of your foot matches the widest part of a size-eleven shoe. If you purchase a size-ten shoe, for example, the widest part of the foot now gets jammed into the upper regions of the size ten, where it has already begun to taper. Not an ideal fit! And believe me, the heel-to-ball measurement is often different from the heel-to-toe measurement. Once you discover your heel-to-ball measurement with the Brannock device, you are well on your way to choosing a shoe that actually fits your foot.

STEP 3

Always buy shoes with removable inserts. This provides you with more foot-care options and usually indicates a higher technical grade of shoe.

One of the neatest tricks I've discovered—to get some sense of whether the shoe fits—is to take both sets of inserts out and stand on them. The inserts represent how much room you have inside of the shoe. Make sure that the inserts completely surround your foot. You do not want your foot extending over the front of the insert or hanging over the sides. As you will discover in the next step, make sure you have enough room up front.

Step 4

Have a thumbs-width distance between your toes and the front of the shoe. Gauge this distance by placing your thumb perpendicular to the top of your big toe as you stand on the removable insert. There should be enough room above the big toe to allow you to place your thumb (widthwise) on the insert without your thumb falling off. The only exception to this rule pertains to those of you (like me) who have what is often called a Morton's toe—a condition where the second toe is longer than the big toe. Morton's toes are fairly common and mean that you must apply the thumb test to the space above the second toe as well as the first.

Phil Maffetone once shared with me his ultimate strategy for finding the right pair of shoes. Go into the store and keep increasing the size by half-size increments until you get a pair that is absolutely hysterically too big—the kind of absurd fit that makes your feet look like they belong to a clown. He claims that the right size for you is the pair you put on just before them.

Step 5

Make sure you have sufficient width in the toe box. This step is actually related to steps two and three. I repeat it here if only to emphasize how important it is that your shoe accommodate the width of your foot across its widest span, which is the ball. I have noticed that certain shoe companies tend to make shoes with narrower toe boxes than others. Whether you have narrow or wide feet, take care to ensure that the foot is able to spread out. Having a wide enough toe box is as important as choosing the proper length. If there is pressure against the side of your foot, the foot can arch up side-to-side and create severe discomfort underneath the ball of your foot, a condition called dropped metatarsal heads.

Try this: take your left hand and place it over your right hand. Place your hands so that the palm of your left hand is above the base of your right thumb and the fingers of your left hand are hanging over the right side of your right hand just below your pinky finger. Now squeeze your right hand with your left. This side-to-side pressure can cause the knuckles on your right hand to arch up. Now imagine the same kind of lateral pressure on your feet, the kind of pressure that gets exerted when the toe-box area is too narrow. Instead of your knuckles being forced into this archlike position, the metatarsal heads (aka the knuckles in your feet) are. This is a compromising position for your feet to be in. Your body weight cannot be supported indefinitely in this position. Eventually, the metatarsal heads drop to fill in the space underneath the arch created by the pressure of the narrow toe box walls. This condition can be painful, and I have seen it a lot. In fact, I used to get it a lot, but not since I purchased shoes with a wide enough toe box (in my case, a "4EEEE" width).

STEP 6

Match the structure and function of your foot to the shape and style of the shoe. The array of running shoes in a store can be overwhelming, especially with shoe styles changing every few months. Salespeople can be helpful, but ideally you should know enough about your own feet to choose the best shoe. Also, knowing your foot characteristics can enable you to use search engines on the Internet that allow you to plug in your foot type and a model of shoe is selected based on the information provided.

The most important considerations to make when it comes to the structure and function of your foot have to do with the following:

- arch type
- tilt pattern
- foot strike

The arch type

This means your foot can have a high arch, low arch, or somewhere in between (medium arch). You can identify your arch type by performing a home version of the imprinter test described earlier.

Bare your feet and have some water and a few sheets of legal-size absorbent paper handy. Place the absorbent paper on the floor in front of you. Get one foot wet at a time, and then step on the absorbent paper with as natural a walking gait as possible. Look straight ahead and keep your arms swinging comfortably by your side. Check the pattern of the water stain left by your foot on the absorbent paper. If the water print left by your foot consists of nearly two distinct marks, one for your heel and one for your forefoot—with only a narrow ridge connecting the two—then you have a high arch. If, on the other hand, the area between your heel and forefoot is almost completely filled in, as if your entire foot were flush against the paper as you took a step, then you can conclude you have a low arch or flat foot (like me). If the water image is somewhere in between, you probably have a medium arch.

Many models of shoes are identified as being best suited for a particular arch type. Knowing your arch type can be helpful in shoe selection. As people age, there seems to be a tendency for some of the elasticity in the foot to be lost, causing a natural age-related dropping of the arch. I generally recommend that everyone consider a medical-grade arch support, regardless of the arch type, although I am aware that there are some highly respected health practitioners who don't agree with me. I do not know of a single commercially available shoe that provides a medical-grade arch support. The inserts that come with most off-the-shelf shoes are really more cosmetic than corrective or supportive in nature. When adding an arch support, check with the manufacturer or your health practitioner about whether to remove the inserts that came with the shoes.

I first started using an orthotic insert in 1983 as I was preparing to compete in the La Rochelle six-day race. All the runners in this prestigious race faced one major obstacle: the course consists of an indoor 200-meter *cement* oval track! This unforgiving surface requires runners either to adopt an easy gliding shuffle or to risk injury. Power running leads to inevitable breakdowns. In hope of reducing stress from the constant pounding, all the competitors covet footgear that can provide ample arch support, cushioning, and shock absorption. I knew going in that successfully dealing with this challenge could determine the eventual winner. After much research I decided to use an orthotic support. There are many high-quality prefabricated and customized orthotic management systems available. Some of the more well-known ones are C.F.M. Orthotic, Universal Pedorthic Services, Apex Foot Health Industries, and Power Point by JM Enterprises. I chose a pair of prefabricated orthotics called Lynco Biomechanical Orthotic Systems manufactured by Dick Schwartz's company, APEX. The inserts offered medical-grade support and cushioning that had a tremendous effect on my ability to tame this ruthless surface. I eventually set a new American record in that event, running 571 miles over six consecutive days, and have been using and recommending the inserts ever since.

I am sure that whichever high-quality orthotic management systems you choose you will be pleased. The American College of Sports Medicine published a study showing that of the 350 runners with common running ailments, 75 percent reported complete resolution or great improvement with the use of orthotics. Some 90 percent of the runners continued to use the orthotic devices even after resolution of their symptoms.

Using an orthotic system can lessen the importance of matching your arch type with a particular style of shoe. However, what might be even more significant is matching the tilt of the foot to the "last" of the shoe.

The tilt pattern

This refers to what is often called the pattern of pronation or supination. The pronator displays an inward tilt of the foot and directs energy and bears weight toward the inside or medial aspects of the foot. The supinator exhibits an opposite pattern. When a person supinates, the foot tilts outward and the energy and weight bearing is diverted to the outside or lateral region of the foot.

The procedure for identifying the tilt of your foot is relatively easy, but you'll need a partner. Observe the manner in which each of you walks. The procedure is simple. Stand behind your partner. Ask your partner to walk straight ahead, arms hanging comfortably by the side. Focus on the ankle. Notice the stability or lack thereof in the ankle. If your partner's ankle seems to tilt inward, toward the midline (medial) side of the body, then he is pronating. Conversely, if your partner's ankle seems to tilt outward toward the outside (lateral) side of the body, then he is supinating. If the ankle remains is fairly upright and stable, then the pattern can be described as "even."

Pronators benefit from shoes that promote stability and motion control. Shoes that have this capability are termed straight lasted.

A straight-lasted shoe can be identified by looking at the shape of the sole—technically called the last shape. The last can have a variety of shapes. The most noticeable changes in last design have to do with the contour of the instep or medial aspect of the shoe (the side that faces the midline of the body). The straighter the medial aspect of the shoe last, the more stability is provided. Having the inside edge of the shoe straight can be quite beneficial for a pronator, since the pronator ends up bearing most of his or her body weight towards the inside of the foot.

The need to purchase a straight-lasted shoe is less pronounced for the supinator. Since the supinator directs his weight toward the outside (lateral aspect) of the foot, the added stability provided by the straighter instep does not have the same positive impact. The supinator has the option of selecting a more curved-lasted shoe. The curved-lasted shoe is marked by the more pronounced bend in the shape of the instep.

The foot strike

This refers to either: (a) the degree to which the foot rotates left-to-right as it makes contact with the ground, or (b) whether the initial contact with the ground is made with the heel or forefoot.

Did you ever notice how some people walk or run with their feet pointed out—duck-footed, as my kids call it—while others end up with their toes pointing in, toward each other—what my kids call pigeon-toed?

If it is not obvious to you what your foot strike pattern is, perform a simple jump test. Just stand comfortably with your weight evenly distributed left-to-right. Close your eyes. Let your arms hang by your side. Now bend your knees slightly and jump about six inches off the ground three consecutive times. When you are done, hold your position. Then, open your eyes and look down. The position your feet end up with is probably a fairly good representation of the rotation of your strike pattern.

All of the walking and the vast majority of the endurance running to be described in this book will emphasize a heel strike or heel placement. More specifically, the initial contact with the ground is usually the outer region of the heel, with the body weight shifting forward as the foot completes it motion during a typical walking/running gait.

There are occasions, however, when the initial foot placement changes. Sprinting, or very fast running (I call this flight-or-fight running), shifts the body weight forward and toward the front of the foot. This typically results in a strike pattern that is called a forefoot strike. For sprinters and forefoot strikers, a stable heel or even straight last shoe is of little consequence. I counsel runners other than sprinters on the value and long-term benefit of a more heel-to-toe style of running. We will explore this issue in depth later.

There can be a relationship between the arch type, tilt pattern, and foot strike. A common combination is a low-arched, heel-striking pronator with an outward rotation of the foot. Another common pattern is the high-arched, forefoot-striking supinator with an inward rotation of the foot. While these patterns may tend to be the most common, there certainly can be other permutations. Who knows, there must assuredly be some medium-arched, nontilting, forefoot-striking even striders or a high-arched, heel-striking pronator with inward stride. The key is to match the structure and function of the foot to the shape and style of the shoe. Once you have identified your arch type, tilt pattern, and foot strike, you can select the model that will work best for you.

STEP 7

Use muscle testing to assess the fit of the shoe. There are muscle-testing techniques that you could use to see if your muscles get strengthened or weakened when you wear a pair of orthotics. While in the shoe store, perform the basic muscle-testing technique:

extend your arm perpendicular to your body, and have someone apply pressure on the back of your outstretched hand while you stand with no shoes on. This test will be your benchmark. Next, try on the shoe model, and walk around the store or run around the block. Use the muscle-testing technique again to determine if your body is strengthened or weakened by the particular shoe.

Given the fluidity of the shoe industry, I will not recommend particular models. The model I might recommend now could be outdated or discontinued by the time the book is published. There are some spectacular services on the Internet that can help you match up arch type, tilt pattern, and foot strike with a specific model. One of the best is the "shoe dog," available from www.roadrunner-sports.com. You can also link up with almost any major shoe manufacturer's home page to receive referrals for running and walking shoes based on your particular needs. Then, there is always the neighborhood sporting-goods outlet or nationwide chain store. Now you are armed with the essential strategies that will empower you to make the best choice for you.

Shoe Wear—What Does It Tell You?

Some people attribute much importance to examining the wear patterns of shoes. While this is a common practice, I do not place as much significance on the wear pattern as I do on the examination of the arch, tilt, and strike pattern. However there is some interesting information to be derived, so let's take a look.

EXAMINING THE SOLE OF THE SHOE (OR SHOE LAST)

Because of the normal biomechanics of the foot in a walking/jogging/distance-running motion, the lateral aspect of the heel (outside) usually makes the initial contact with the ground and bears most of the weight. Outer-heel wear pattern is fairly common. If, on the other hand, inner-heel wear is significant, this might be an indication that the walker/runner is a severe pronator. But, again, observing the tilt of the foot as a person moves is probably the best indicator of whether a person pronates.

Forefoot wear with little or no erosion of the heel can be a sign of a forefoot striker. This is more common for sprinters and some middle-distance runners, described earlier, who tend to run at faster paces.

Excessive wear along the outside (lateral aspect) of the shoe may indicate a high arch, excessively supinating foot. Excessive wear along the inside (medial aspect) of the shoe probably indicates severe and excessive pronation.

EXAMINING THE SHOE BOX OR UPPER

As you accumulate miles, your foot will create a distinct imprint in your shoe. Look in the upper portion of the shoe for the tilt of the shoe box. As in observing a person's gait, an inward tilt of the upper can reveal a severe pronation pattern, while an outward tilt can mean excessive supination.

Another area to focus on is the integrity of the shoe box itself. Are there holes by the toes? This usually means the shoe is too short. As we learned earlier, there should be at least a thumb's width distance between your toes and the front of the shoe.

Assessing the wear pattern of the shoe can help you determine when you need a new pair. I follow a simple rule: when the integrity of the shoe is compromised in any way—a hole develops in the toe box, an air pillow collapses, or the bottom layer of the sole wears down to the point where the layer beneath it is exposed—it's time for a change.

Another indicator of the need to buy new shoes is mileage, though individual expectancies vary greatly. Certain practices can extend shoe life considerably. Make sure your shoes fit, and purchase more than one pair of shoes so you can alternate their use. Orthotics, which promote optimal weight distribution, can also ensure that our shoes last longer. I have worn shoes for as long as three months, accumulating approximately a thousand miles. More likely, shoe life expectancy is between three hundred and five hundred miles.

Frequently Asked Questions About Footwear

SHOULD I ROTATE MY SHOES?

If purchasing more than one pair of shoes at a time is an option to you, I highly recommend rotating your shoes. By rotating your shoes, I simply mean that you do not run in the same pair of shoes two days in a row. Give your shoes a chance to breathe, dry out, and recover. This strategy will increase the life of your shoes and could have an impact on the aroma they emit.

IS IT PREFERABLE TO RUN WITH LIGHTER-WEIGHT SHOES?

Just like the misguided tendency to purchase shoes that are too small, most people I meet seem to place way too much emphasis on the weight of the shoe. I personally believe that more emphasis should be placed on finding shoes that fit and less on how much the shoe weighs. Wearing light racing shoes for the bulk of your training or even during longer races of half-marathon or more is not something that I recommend.

A Lot of Shoes Have Pods or Air Pockets— Is This a Recommended Feature?

There is currently a trend toward more and more cushioning in shoes. Try to avoid shoes that are significantly elevated off of the ground. While the addition of added air pillows, shock-absorbing pads, and thicker soles may create the sensation that you are walking on air, there could be a downside. As the height and padding increases, so does the potential for lateral (side-to-side) instability. There is a trade-off between that cushiness and that lateral instability that can effect your joints. I recommend selecting shoes that are more moderate in terms of the height (and price), remove the standard inserts, then add a pair of pre-fabricated orthotics.

I've Spent a Lot on Custom Orthotics, and I Still Have Foot Problems—Why?

Whether or not you chose to use an orthotic insert, the primary focus must be on selecting shoes that fit. The most magnificently constructed orthotic will not work if slipped into shoes that are too small or narrow. No matter what kind of an orthotic you have, if you put them into shoes that don't fit, you're not going to solve the problem.

Even When I Double-Tie My Laces, They Come Undone. Any Suggestions?

Rather than tying your shoelaces conventionally, use a pair of lace locks. I first became exposed to lace locks during my triathlon days, though the technology has been familiar to outdoor adventurers and mountain climber for years.

Lace locks eliminate the need to tie your shoes and allow the adjustment of shoe tension in a matter of moments. Triathletes use lace locks to speed up the changes in the transition areas as they move from event to event and have to change shoes. I first used them because I noticed that after hours upon hours of running I found the simple task of tying my shoes challenging and one I would rather do without.

Lace locks are small cylindrical devices that serve the same function as the convention knotted bow. Pinch the end of the cylinder and a gap opens up in the center through which the shoelaces can be drawn. When you let go of the ends of the lace lock, the center closes, locking the laces in position without the need of a secure knot. Once you begin using lace locks, you'll be amazed how easy it is to get your shoes on or off and how quickly you'll be able to adjust the tension in your shoe so that you make them feel "just right." Lace locks can be purchased at most outdoor stores and specialty shops that service runners or triathletes.

12

Breathe for Maximum Energy

I once asked my close friend Dr. Nate Zinsser, director of the Center for Human Performance at the United States Military Academy, to name the most important technique for getting in touch with the body. His reply was instantaneous: "Become aware of where you are in the breathing cycle."

In my twenties, when I practiced yoga and meditation, breathing was something that was studied rather than taken for granted. In karate we brought heightened awareness to the simple process of breathing. As a runner, I've discovered how breathing can lead to increased energy, productivity, and capacity to endure. The technique that all these physical disciplines advocate is belly breathing.

Belly breathing is used in everything from opera singing to power lifting—the low-to-the-belly method of breathing crosses all physical cultures. Breathing to the belly calms and energizes at the same time.

Have you ever noticed what happens to your breathing when you become anxious or uptight? The shoulder muscles tense, the breathing rises into the chest, and the breath becomes shallow and more rapid. You may recognize this sequence of events when you move into states of uncertainty or alarm—and, as you will learn, when your body begins to shift into a fight-or-flight sugar-burning mode. During such episodes, if someone tells you to calm down or take a deep breath, what he's actually saying is breathe to your belly. Manage your breathing, and you manage your state.

Try this: stand facing a full-length mirror, with your arms hanging comfortably by your sides. Take a deep breath, and keep an eye on what happens to your body. Which part of your body moves first? Is it your shoulders? Your chest? Or does your breath originate in your abdomen or lower abdomen? Repeat the procedure. Breathe in. Hold momentarily and breathe out. Again, which part of your body moved first? Asked a different way—to where did you breathe? Was it your shoulders? Chest? What about your abdomen or lower abdomen?

If you answered shoulders or chest, you need to work on your breathing technique. Try the following exercise. Either stand comfortably with slightly bent knees, feet shoulder-width apart, arms by your side, weight evenly distributed right-to-left side. Or lie on your back with your knees bent and feet flat on the floor. Once you get into one of the two starting positions, place one hand on your navel. As you inhale, count to six and bring your breath into the area beneath your hand. This will cause your hand to rise as your abdomen expands. As you exhale to the count of six, your abdomen will deflate and your hand will return to its original position.

Imagine a triangle formed by your hips and your belly button. Place your hands on your hips. See a triangle in your mind's eye. The top of the triangle is your belly button. The sides flare down and back to the outside of your body, toward where your hands rest on your hips. The line that connects the place where your hands are forms the base of the triangle. Imagine a "ball" encased inside this triangle. As you breathe in, see yourself filling the "ball" up with air. As you inhale, the "ball" inflates. It gets larger, becomes more voluminous, expansive, and lighter. As you exhale, the air releases, the "ball" deflates, air flows out, and pressure is released. Breathe in, the "ball" gets bigger. Breathe out, the "ball" gets smaller.

Notice the feeling that begins to envelop you. Chances are you feel more relaxed and peaceful. You are gaining control, connecting to your body. Life's little challenges don't seem as overwhelming or unmanageable. Confidence rises. You are more focused. Energized. Ready to take on whatever comes your way. Breathe to the "ball." Feel the "ball" expand as you breathe in; release air as you breathe out. Take a few deep, diaphragmatic belly breaths and feel what happens.

This concept is challenging to many. We are products of a chest-out, stomach-in culture. I tried the exercise I just described when I was a guest on Regis Philbin's cable-TV talk show. Like most people, Regis took a deep breath and his chest expanded and his shoulders rose up.

Try it out on your friends and family, and you will probably get a similar result. But most children won't fall for it, especially young ones. Take a moment to watch how babies or young children breathe as they sleep. Their little chests and shoulders remain motionless. The entire breathing motion emanates from the belly. I guess babies and young children aren't as self-conscious about their stomachs as we adults are. Most of us are uncomfortable directing attention to our stomachs. If someone does, it is more likely because she has a flat and chiseled stomach than because she has a relaxed and highly developed breathing style.

Whether you're on the way to catch a bus, getting ready for a meeting, or enjoying a comfortable, aerobic run, be aware of where you are in the breathing cycle and whether you're breathing lower to your belly or higher to your chest.

To maximize your endurance, you want to breathe deeply to your belly, to the "ball" inside the triangle formed by your hips and belly button. Do so and you'll release tension throughout your body. Practice your diaphragmatic breathing regularly. Use this technique whenever you begin to feel tense, uptight, anxious, or fatigued. Concentrate on creating a breathing cycle that begins in your lower abdomen to enhance your energy, calm you down, and promote a feeling of health and well-being.

Breathing can be initiated through the mouth or the nose. Master both methods of breathing. Each technique produces a slightly different experience. Nostril breathing creates a sense of energy being released and cleansing. It seems to draw the flow of air up and back as if oxygenating the brain. The flow of breath then moves back and down the spine, working its way behind, below, and finally up into the "ball" encased inside the triangle formed by the hips and belly button.

With mouth breathing, the flow of air travels directly down along the front of the body to the "ball." When you breathe through the mouth, you're breathing straight to the "ball."

As you run, discover which breathing strategy feels most comfortable to you. Be aware of the distinctions you create by breathing one way or another. At low levels of intensity, when not much effort is needed to sustain movement, breathe from either the nose or the mouth. As you increase your intensity, your breathing will shift naturally to the mouth. Mouth breathing delivers a greater volume of air in a shorter amount of time, over a more direct route than nose breathing. Quick bites of air are not possible through the nose.

Be sensitive to this nose-to-mouth breathing change as you gradually increase your effort on a run. Many people who try to force nostril breathing think it's better than mouth breathing. Rather than force the breathing back to the nostril, let it happen naturally. If your body wants to breathe through the mouth, let it. Later on, I will show how to use the location of the breathing as an indicator of whether your body is burning fat or burning sugar. For now though, follow the energy of your body. Go with its natural flow. Accept its innate wisdom.

13

Focus Your Form on a Series of Metaphors

People often ask what I think about when I run for days on end. Sometimes I let random thoughts come into my mind such as what I did yesterday or what I want to do tomorrow. Most of the time, I maintain a conscious connection with my body so I can continue moving forward with a sense of effortlessness, comfort, and natural flow. I concentrate on my breathing, the relationship of my feet to the ground, the position of my arms, my hand, my jaw, and constantly monitor the sights, sounds, and feelings of the world around me. I do not let myself become preoccupied with how much longer I have to go or whether I can push myself harder.

I am able to maintain this state of awareness by employing a series of metaphors. With these metaphors I can transform what I am doing into a motion that feels relatively comfortable, effortless, and flowing. I'd like to share them with you right now. Rather than running as hard as you can, the more empowering strategy is to continually reference these metaphors as you move. The point isn't how quickly you can go or how much pain you can take in order to speed up. Running faster doesn't have to mean working harder. While this approach might work for a sprint, your body won't stand for it over the course of many miles. Maintaining the metaphors will take you away from obsessing about the outcome and instead bring you deeper into the process of moving, enriching both your experience and your progress.

I am on my second training run with a client, and afterward we return to my office to assess how he's doing. He talks excitedly about the running metaphors. He says they're life-changing—not only for him, but for his eight-year-old son. He shares that his son was having trouble keeping up with the kids in his gym class during group runs. He would push and push, becoming so exhausted and out of breath he could never move up from the rear of the pack. After our initial run/walk analysis session, my client went home and shared with his son many of the new distinctions he picked up from me. Instead of trying to run faster, my client's son began concentrating on the series of metaphors his dad passed along. By changing his focus, his son began to relax, getting into the flow of movement, and avoided the pain and discomfort he previously experienced. He came home that day, excitedly sharing the news with his father that during the day's group run, he ended up in the middle of the pack. When my client passes the story on to me, it reinforces my belief in the power of the metaphors.

Movement Metaphor 1: Breathing

BREATHE TO THE "BALL" FORMED BY YOUR HIPS AND BELLY BUTTON

Your breath is the glue that connects the mind and the body. As you run, notice where you are in the breathing cycle. Awareness of where you are in the breathing cycle integrates the mind and the body. Breathe low and to the belly. With each breath imagine a triangle formed by your hips and your belly button. Inside of the triangle is a "ball." As you breathe in, fill the "ball" with air. As you breathe out, feel the air escape as the "ball" becomes smaller.

Exercise:

When you run, from time to time place your hand over your belly button. As you breathe in, feel the "ball" expand as it gently pushes your hand outward. Exhale and feel the air slowly escape from the "ball" as your hand moves inward. Become attuned to the powerful sensation of being energized from the center of your body outward.

Movement Metaphor 2: Foot Position

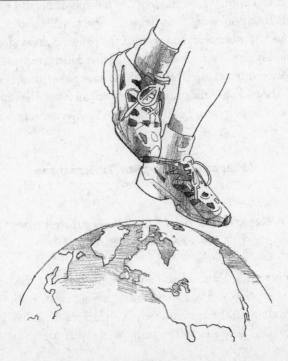

LIFT YOUR FEET UP JUST ENOUGH TO
LET THE EARTH PASS BENEATH YOU

Imagine you're standing on the top of the world as it is rotating. With each step, all you are doing is lifting your feet up just enough to let the earth pass beneath you. Imagine everything is flowing toward you as though you're on a giant treadmill. You're not going anywhere; everything in the world is coming toward you. Like scenery of an old movie, the background is always moving, and you are staying in the same place. Energy flows from the back of the foot to the front of the foot. With each step feel the energy move down your spine to the heel of your foot, over the arch, and out your toes. Let your heel be the first part of your body that makes contact with the ground. Feel your body weight being supported by your heel. Let your body weight shift forward over the arch of your foot to the front of your foot. Feel your heel lift off the ground as your body weight shifts forward to the ball of your foot and your toes spread out. Finally your entire foot lifts up off the ground just enough to let the earth pass beneath. Change your perception from pushing down on the ground to lifting your feet up off the ground. Remember, the earth is moving. It is always moving. All you are doing is lifting your feet up just enough to let it pass beneath.

Exercise:

As you move, appreciate the sense of flow and momentum that is inherent in the heel-to-ball movement of the foot. Start off by walking comfortably with your arms by your side, emphasizing the heel-to-ball movement described above. Feel your body weight shifting from the back of your foot to the front of your foot. Feel the energy flow from the back to the front. Sense the movement of the earth beneath you, the constant momentum of the rotation of the earth.

Now shift the placement of your feet, and begin walking on your toes, letting the front of your foot make contact with the ground first. Notice how the sense of movement and flow is replaced by a staccato feeling of starting and stopping. Energy no longer moves down your back through the rear of the foot over the arch to the front of your foot and out your toes. Instead, energy seems to collect in the front of your foot, getting sent backward through your ankle and ending up in your calf. The tension in your calf becomes noticeable; your ankles become unstable; you have to exert effort to stabilize your body and keep yourself upright.

Now change again so that instead of walking on the front of your foot, you walk flat-footed. Your entire foot makes contact with the ground at the same time. Notice that the tightness in your calf is released and stability returns to your ankles. However, now you feel subtle vibrations as energy flows down your body to the ground and ricochets back up your body. The sense of momentum, while different from front-foot walking, is still not the same as when you first began. There is still a starting-and-stopping feel to the movement. The treadmill-like sensation is still absent.

When you shift back to the heel-to-ball motion, you almost immediately sense the return of stability and momentum. Your body calms down, the vibrations disappear, and the treadmill effect returns.

Movement Metaphor 3: Upper-Body Position

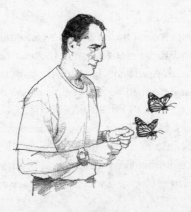

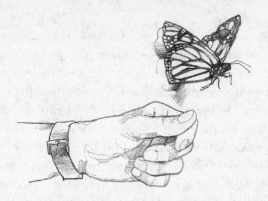

MOVE WITH DINOSAUR ARMS
HOLDING BUTTERFLIES

As you move, bring your arms up into dinosaur arm position. Picture a dinosaur, a Tyrannosaurus Rex, with tiny little arms that remain bent at the elbows. This is the position you want your arms to be in.

Continue moving—elbows bent, wrists above your elbows, and arms pressed ever so slightly against your body, the way they would be if you tucked a newspaper under each armpit. Apply the right amount of pressure to keep the imaginary newspaper in position, but not so much as to crumple the pages. As you move with your T-Rex arms, keep the newspaper in place.

Next imagine you're holding a butterfly in each hand. Your hands are closed around the butterfly just enough to keep them from flying away. Relax your hands enough so that the butterfly has enough room to flutter its wings. Feel the wings of the butterfly fluttering on the inside of your hands. Turn your palms so that they face each other as you move holding butterflies in your dinosaur arms.

Exercise:

Moving at a comfortable pace, bring your arms up to the dinosaur position. Feel the wings of the butterfly fluttering on the inside of your hands as you move. Feel the energy flow as your body moves through time and space. Release the butterflies, let your arms fall to your sides, and notice how your energy seems to drop and your sense of synchronicity seems to disappear. Continue moving with your arms by your side. Feel the disappearance of the synchronicity that you maintained in the dinosaur position. The energy drops and your sense of momentum slows down. It's as though the arms-up position keep the energy in and the arms-down position lets the energy out. Notice the change in how you feel. When the arms drop to your sides, your sense of movement becomes sluggish. You probably want to move more slowly.

As someone who has run for all these years and all these miles, I'm still amazed at the remarkable change that such a subtle shift in body position can bring about. I can explain it in terms of the different muscles it engages. With the arms up, the body relies more on the large muscles of the back and chest than the smaller muscles of the biceps and triceps.

But part of me is content with the belief that the energy shift is brought about by the magic of the metaphor. If I'm ever feeling down or out of rhythm, I remind myself to feel the butterflies in my hands as I move with dinosaur arms, and I am suddenly back in the flow.

Movement Metaphor 4: Head Position

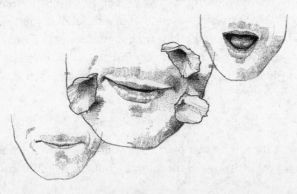

HOLD ROSE PETALS IN THE CORNER OF YOUR MOUTH

Position your mouth as though you are holding a rose petal in each corner. Hold the petals in the corner of your mouth by turning your lips slightly upward. Exert just enough pressure to keep the rose petals in place but not enough to crush them. You want to feel a sense of relaxed control.

Exercise:

Scrunch your face. Grind your teeth tightly. Hold this position for a few seconds. Would you like to run with this much stress? No way! Go in the opposite direction, and try to keep your mouth open as you run. Note the distinction between the clenched jaw and running with your mouth open wide. Both positions create stress in your jaw. Find a position somewhere in between, and the best way to do it is to run with rose petals in the corner of your mouth.

Movement Metaphor 5: Eye Position

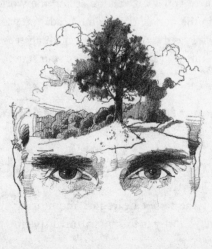

Distinguish "Hard Eyes" from "Soft Eyes"

Sometimes a simple shift from "hard eyes" to "soft eyes" can create a change in state that will empower you to continue moving forward with the greatest of ease. To assume the hard-eye position, focus on a spot in front of you. Look ahead through the center of your eye with a laser-beam focus. Try making the edges of whatever you're looking at as distinct and sharp as possible.

Next, shift to soft eyes by putting images slightly out of focus. Look ahead as though you're taking in the world through the center of your forehead. You're not looking at anything in particular but everything at once.

Exercise:

Identify a point ahead of you, perhaps a tree. Imagine your vision is like a laser beam moving from the middle of your eye to the outline of the tree. Make your focus strong and clear, so that the edges of the tree are hard and distinct, completely in focus, and in the center of your field of vision. Now, put all the images in front of you slightly out of focus. Avoid looking at any one object in particular. Take in all the scenery in front of you, as if you are seeing the world through an imaginary eye in the middle of your forehead. You want the view to be soft and flowing, as if you are seeing everything at once. The point is to be able to shift your focus and change your state.

Movement Metaphor 6: State Maintenance

Run As Though You Are on a Roller Coaster

The point of the target heart-rate monitoring strategies that will be explained shortly is to stay within a specific training zone on any given day. In order to do so, adopt the metaphor of the roller coaster. As the roller coaster moves up and down hills, it gains momentum going downhill and loses momentum going uphill. If you attempt to maintain the same pace going up and down hills, it's certain you will have to work much harder going up the hill than going down. Trying to maintain a steady pace defeats the purpose of using a heart-rate monitor. It's not how fast you're going uphill, but how well you master maintaining the same state as you move. The roller-coaster metaphor challenges you to be in touch with your body as you manage each moment. The goal is to make the necessary adjustments so that you remain at the same comfort level throughout the movement session.

Exercise:

The best way to maintain your target zone as you're moving up and down hills is to make changes in the length of your stride. As you approach a hill, pretend you're the roller coaster and let yourself lose momentum by slowing down as you move up the hill. You do this by taking small steps, baby steps, as small as the size of your feet. Notice how the effort level seems to remain constant. You no longer have to work harder to get up the hill. The hills begin to disappear. As you come over the crest of the hill, like a roller coaster, let yourself gain momentum coming down. Without forcing yourself to run faster, just increase the length of your stride so you cover more ground with each step. Go with the flow of gravity as it pulls you down the hill. As you reach level ground, let your foot stride shorten and return to normal.

Movement Metaphor 7: Making Adjustments

IMAGINE YOURSELF AS CAPTAIN OF A SHIP

When the time comes for you to implement your training program, you'll be asked to stay in a target heart-rate zone that I will recommend to you. There will be times when your heart rate will go above or below the recommended zone, requiring you to either pick up the pace or slow down. You want to make these adjustments as though you're the captain of a ship rather than the driver of a car. As the captain of a ship, you must make subtle changes—if you accelerate or decelerate too quickly, you'll lose control of the ship. Unlike the car driver, who can accelerate quickly and stop suddenly, the ship's captain must anticipate changes and implement them in a controlled manner.

Your objective is to regularly visit these metaphors as you move. Reconnect with your breathing. Revisit your relationship to the ground. With each step feel your body being supported by the heel as your foot makes a continuous heel-to-ball motion. Imagine the earth rotating beneath you. Feel your arms ever so slightly brushing against the sides of your body as they keep the newspaper in place. Be aware of the sensation of the wings of the butterflies fluttering on the inside of your hands. Feel the rose petals that you're holding in the corners of your mouth. Shift from hard eyes to soft eyes and back again.

These metaphors can generate an effective, efficient, and effortless style of movement. Sometimes, you may be running through a rough patch and simply going through the series of metaphors can pull you out. At the very worst, if the metaphors don't pull you out of the bad patch, after you go through the inventory you'll be five minutes farther along than when you started.

14

Discover the Appeal of Burning Fat

For a long time I believed that it didn't matter where your body got its energy. You could burn sugar or you could burn fat. Your body relied on sugar when it needed immediate and considerable energy. It switched over to fat when sugar stores began to run out or if the task at hand was relatively easy. As long as there was fuel available to burn, what difference did it make if it was fat or sugar? That is what I learned in school, and it is the belief held by most athletes. But my experience has taught me to question conventional wisdom. Through my extensive training and exposure to alternative-health practitioners, I've become convinced that it does matter where your body gets its energy. There is a difference between burning fat and burning sugar. While your body can burn either fuel, it is far better off burning fat. Fat is the body's fuel of choice. Fat, not sugar, is our most inexhaustible and healthful energy resource.

I say this in the face of a society intent on burning sugar for energy. Most people rely too much on sugar for the quick boost. As a culture we have become addicted to sugar. Nowhere is this more pronounced than in the running world. The night before the New

York City Marathon, when I went to dinner with a local television celebrity with whom I was training, an elderly couple sitting next to us reminded us to "get those carbs in" by eating plenty of pasta. Like the majority of the population, they were certain the best way to prepare was to load up on sugar stores. Later the next day, the streets of New York were paved with empty packets of sugary gels.

While sugar-based energy is fast and effective, it has long-term drawbacks, chiefly inconsistent energy levels and making the body more acidic, which could increase your susceptibility to colds, flus, and injuries. The long term does matter! What prevents most people from maintaining and enjoying a lifetime exercise program is their reliance on sugar-based energy.

The next chapter deals with how to organize your training around burning fat, and in the "Eat for the Distance" section you'll learn which foods are best for fat-burning. For now, I want you to understand why you must avoid sugar as an energy source and instead train your body to become a fat-burning machine.

The human body has two distinct energy-producing systems: one is based on burning sugar, generally referred to as the anaerobic system; the other based on fat, or the aerobic system. The sugar-based anaerobic system evolved to fuel the fight-or-flight response. Throughout evolution we have relied on sugar-based fuel for survival. Our ancestors tapped into it to run from—or run after—other animals. Anaerobic energy is an emergency system, designed to quickly mobilize energy to flee, defend yourself, or be the aggressor when your life is threatened. The problem today is that we put ourselves in sugar-burning states all the time. This instant energy comes at a price.

To begin with, your body does not have a lot of sugar to use as energy. Of the approximately 160,000 calories stored in the body, only about 2,500 come from sugar (23,000 are protein; 134,500 are from fat). By developing a dependency on sugar-based energy, you place your fate in the hands of a finite and scarce fuel source. Also, it's stressful for your body to produce energy by burning sugar. The by-products of sugar metabolism can impair your ability to be strong and optimistic in the long run of life.

By design the day-to-day function of your sugar-based energy system is to fuel the nervous system and brain and provide energy in case of an emergency. Now if you go out for a long, fast run without a fat-mobilizing warmup, your body immediately taps into its sugar stores to provide energy for you to move. So when the amount of sugar in your body begins to drop, it sends you warning signals: loss of concentration, dizziness, lack of coordination, and, in extreme cases, blurry vision. Most of us interpret these symptoms as signs that our body is running out of energy and that we need more fuel. In reality these are warning signals that the body knows its emergency fuel supply is being depleted and that it can no longer protect itself. The only answer is to stop moving or to take in an exogenous energy source: carbohydrates (all carbohydrates are eventually broken down to sugar), an energy bar, or a sugary energy-replacement drink. Thus, a vicious circle begins. Your blood sugar level rises and falls with every change in your training and diet. When your blood sugar drops, so does your ability to keep moving. You become prone to injuries, fatigue, and mood swings. My greatest revelation in this area occurred in late summer, 1984.

I am invited to La Rochelle, France, for the premier six-day race. As the only American among a cadre of multiday ultramarathon specialists, I train hard for a great performance. One month before I am set to leave, I arrive at my last scheduled race before La Rochelle. It is a highly publicized triathlon on Long Island, New York. I am not feeling great, though. For the past several months, an irritation on my right foot has grown from an annoyance to a full-blown incapacitating injury. A lump the size of a ping-pong ball has emerged on my right foot, midway between my little toe and ankle. It is tender to the touch and sends piercing spikes of pain through my body when I try to run.

The day before the race, I go to Ray Charron, a close friend who happens to be the race director, to tell him I have to drop out. Ray says he understands, but asks me to indulge him with one favor beforehand. He suggests I see a chiropractor, Philip Maffetone, who is at the event with another athlete. I have already seen nearly a dozen medical doctors, chiropractors, and bodyworkers and have basically given up hope that my injury can be fixed. But Phil has a reputation for getting broken down, over-trained, world-class athletes back up and running, so I agree.

I am introduced to Phil at the VFW Hall. Tall and lanky, with a shock of curly white hair, Phil is soft spoken and thoughtful. He has the presence of a true healer. He takes me to a clearing outside of the registration area and asks me to lie down on the grass. He begins testing my muscles, having me resist as he applies pressure to my arms and legs. Familiar with muscle testing methodologies, I know Phil is trying to get information about my body by testing the strength and weakness of certain indicator muscles.

After a few minutes, he stops and places his hands around my ailing foot. "Relax" he says. Suddenly he snaps my foot, and the lump disappears!

Noticing the shocked expression on my face, he responds, "This is just first aid. If you really want me to help you, you need to make changes in how you train and what you eat." Phil explains that the discomfort I am experiencing is related to a number of factors, including "anaerobic excess." I have been training and eating in such a way as to turn my body into a sugar-burning, fat-storing monstrosity. This exaggerated reliance on sugar has stressed my body and caused the injury. "The point of your training isn't to see how fast you can get your feet to move," Phil says. "The point is to get your body to change the way it gets energy. You want it to burn more fat and less sugar."

Phil believes that the stress of burning sugar has affected the way my body functions. My body weight was not being evenly distributed through my skeletal system. Instead of stress flowing down and out my body, it flowed down and to the right, putting pressure on my foot and dislodging a bone. An unstable bone may have created the pain, but the imbalance that caused it was based on my body's excessive use of sugar as an energy source.

After Phil's magical "snap," for the first time in months I am able to run a race, in this case a triathlon, without pain, running past marathon legend Allison Roe in the last few hundred yards to place in the top twenty. Now I am ready to prepare for La Rochelle. For the three weeks, I commit to cutting out all sugar. This was more of a challenge than the six-day race. I am like a reformed junkie, constantly battling the urge to experience just one more sugar high. Even during the six-day race it affects me. I circle the indoor track in La Rochelle, gazing longingly at the cookies, cakes, and candies that other runners have spread out across their tables. I even collect a few and stash them in the back of the track, behind a curtain where Phil can't see them. My plan is to sneak a few bites now and again when he isn't looking, but I never do. I stick with the plan. I realize the struggle is worth it. My energy is stronger and noticeably more consistent. I finish in second place, setting a new American record by covering 571 miles in six days.

Upon returning from my remarkable experience in La Rochelle, I enthusiastically change my training to focus on burning fat, not sugar. I allocate more time to training in moderate intensities for longer periods of time. Walking (yech!) becomes part of my regular routine. Given my competitive nature, it is hard to adjust to walking, but over time I come to enjoy it. Phil introduces me to a heart-rate monitor.

Using the heart-rate monitor, we identify my fat-burning zones and make sure I train in them several days a week. In these zones, my breathing is low to the belly and noticeably quiet. Breathing in can occur easily either through the nose or mouth. The sensation is one of comfort and moderation. Thoughts drift and wander. Perception moves easily between internal thoughts and taking in the external world. I can daydream or simply look, listen, and feel what is going on in the world. The visual world has depth and three-dimensionality; it is expansive, with a noticeable peripheral vastness.

Speed workouts in my sugar-burning zone is an entirely different experience. Breathing tends to be exclusively through the mouth, as if that is the only way to get enough air into my body to keep it moving. It rises into my chest and becomes shallow and more rapid. My chest starts to feel tight and constrained. The sound of the forced expulsion of air begins to overwhelm all other sounds, save for the sound of my feet hitting the ground or that little voice inside my head screaming, "Keep running . . . don't let anyone catch you . . . you're almost there!" Perception "tunnels" inward as the visual world flattens out, and the depth and three-dimensionality of the world diminishes. My attention gets drawn into a smaller and smaller area of vision, usually right in front of me and angled slightly down. A growing sense of urgency and alarm replaces that calm and effortless feeling of the fat-burning zone. The focus shifts from feeling well and moving in a comfortable state to an urgent attempt to get through the workout. Instead of feeling a desire to process the sights, sounds, and feelings my body is experiencing, I can't wait for the workout to end. If I do feel satisfaction, it comes from the realization that I am doing something impressive either to me or to people who I think are watching, or that when the session is over I can savor the gratification of a job well done.

From that point on, the sugar-burning/fat-burning distinction became the central feature of my own training philosophies. Your body can burn fat, and your body can burn sugar. If you really want to go the distance, you are infinitely better off burning fat.

When I present this concept in seminars, what often comes to the surface are common myths about fat and sugar-burning, which I'd like to take a moment to dispel here.

Myth
The method that generates results the fastest is the best.

Reality
The more gradual the change, the more likely it will last.

My doctoral advisor at Columbia University once opened his class with the attention-grabbing question: "You want to know the fastest way to lose weight?"

We all sat there ready for a new theory.

"The fastest way to lose weight is to get sick," he told us. "Unfortunately the only way you're guaranteed to keep it off is to die." I know what he means, and probably so do you. The fact that a particular strategy produces results faster does not necessarily mean it is better for you. Yet who can resist the lure of "experts" who claim they have found the secret to fast weight loss in the form of newfangled dietary aids and supplements or instantaneous performance enhancements? While it is tantalizing to discover ways to get results NOW, we must ask such experts, "At what cost?" I usually turn the other way and run when someone approaches me with a new secret formula proven to transform the body overnight. Today we have highly controversial fat substitutes, potentially carcinogenic sugar alternatives, diet pills that cause heart disease, and high intensity-training regimens that offer immediate weight loss—but potentially at the expense of our long-term health and well-being. All of this does not seem too far removed from a bargain with the devil. We all want results—more energy, less weight, and an enhanced performance—and we want it now. Most of us will do anything to get what we want and worry about the consequences later.

I am always wary of using the urgency of performance enhancement and rapidity of change as criteria by which to judge whether or not I will adopt a training or nutritional strategy. Sometimes what gets you there fastest may not be that good for you in the long run. It is better to ask these questions: Will I be more in touch with my body because of it? Will I be healthier, more in balance, more in harmony with my life and the life of those around me? Remind yourself that how you get to your goals and what you do when you finally arrive are at least as important as what the goals are. What good is it if you reach your goal only to find that you cannot hold on to it or that in your haste to get there you never truly learned to appreciate what the journey meant?

Faster is better is the myth of a culture raised on speed and dependent on sugar. When it comes to your long-term health and well-being, slower may be better, and burning fat—not sugar—is the way to go. It might take you a little longer, but I assure you that you will get there just the same. Once you do, you'll be more likely to maintain the progress that you made and be in a position to keep moving on.

Myth
No pain, no gain. You must suffer to get results.

Reality
Comfort is the key to sustainable growth.

When it comes to performance, most people subscribe to the no pain, no gain philosophy of training. It's the same when people want to lose weight or reduce body fat—they tend to believe they must push to the point of pain and discomfort to get results.

Certainly, you can lose fat by working out hard and burning lots of calories, most of which come from sugar. You can also lose fat by training at a much more comfortable intensity and burning copious amounts of fat. Either strategy can cause a loss in body fat. The truth is, though, you can accelerate both short-term weight loss and performance enhancement by repeatedly pushing yourself to the brink of exhaustion then pulling back, recovering, and repeating the cycle for as long and as hard as you can. Combine it with a highly restrictive diet that provides just enough calories to keep you going and you will see results in just a few days.

There is a cost to this frenzied flight-or-fight state. While burning sugar can lead to a reduction of body fat, the stress it creates can have an adverse effect on other systems of the body. When I was a high school and collegiate wrestler, I adhered to a fast-results sugar-burning training strategy, virtually starving myself and then training until I was physically unable to do one more drill. The strategy works, for a while, but it completely ignores the emotional and biochemical terror that it rains on your mood, adrenal glands, nervous system, immune system, and musculoskeletal system. It is one thing to want results now. It is another to sacrifice your health over it.

Constantly working out hard and burning sugar may get you results faster, but it can also move you one step farther away from realizing your inherent power. The no pain, no gain way of being can limit your potential for steady, sustainable, and never-ending forward momentum. If being unstoppable and relentless is important to you, then allow for generous amounts of comfortable fat-burning movement in your life.

Myth
Either you're born to burn fat or you're not.

Reality
You can train your body to burn more fat.

It is true: genes play a role in how likely your body is to utilize fat as an energy source. Each of us inherits a certain proportion of muscle fibers; some are designed to burn fat and others to burn sugar. If you are born with a lot of fat-burning muscle fibers, your body will likely get its energy from fat. The converse is true: inherit a large proportion of sugar-burning muscle fibers, and your body will probably burn more sugar. While we all may be born with a certain ratio of fat-burning to sugar-burning muscle fibers, we can influence how our body uses its energy resources.

Let's start with some basic definitions: Fat-burning muscle fibers are aerobic or "slow-twitch," and sugar-burning fibers are anaerobic or "fast-twitch." Aerobic slow-twitch muscle fibers are relatively slow at producing energy, whereas the anaerobic fast-twitch fibers produce energy rapidly. Most of us are born with slightly more aerobic, slow-twitch, fat-burning muscle fibers. The rest of our inherited muscle fiber type is divided between two types of anaerobic fast-twitch sugar-burning fibers: Type A and Type B. Type B accounts for the smallest percentage, about 13 percent, and are incredibly explosive yet easily fatigued. The remaining muscle fibers are Type A. These muscle fibers are also fast-twitch, but with some added stamina.

While it is impossible to change our inherited proportion of fat-burning to sugar-burning muscle fibers, we can use physical training to transform how our body uses its energy stores. If you perform explosive, all-out sugar-burning exercise such as sprints or high-intensity aerobics, you can increase your muscle fibers' dependency on burning sugar. Whether you actually change a fat-burning muscle fiber into a sugar-burning one or simply increase the size and density of the existing sugar-burning muscles is debatable. In either case, the specific measurable result is that during high-intensity training you draw most of your energy from sugar—not fat. Conversely, when the majority of your training is low to moderate intensity, your body will draw more and more energy from fat. In summary, nice and easy long runs or walks condition your body to rely more on slow-twitch, aerobic, fat-burning muscle fibers, and high-intensity exercise is likely to encourage the stimulation of the powerful sugar-burning ones.

Back to the gene issue, athletes who participate in highly explosive fight-or-flight activities such as sprinting and weight lifting are likely to have higher concentrations of sugar-burning muscle fibers than athletes who participate in moderate-intensity sports such as cross-country skiing and distance running. Sprinters and weight lifters can have as much as 55 percent fast-twitch, sugar-burning muscle fiber. Distance runners and cross-country skiers, on the other hand, have been measured with aerobic fat-burning muscle fiber percentages topping 90 percent. Quite a variation! Keep in mind, however, that part of this documented association may be attributed to the possibility that athletes with a particular muscle fiber makeup are attracted to sports that emphasize their innate attributes.

Still, transformations occur, and they are measurable and demonstrable. Regular exposure to sugar-burning challenges increases the likelihood that you will become even more dependent on sugar as an energy source. Offer your body the chance to burn fat, and it will not only burn fat now, it will be more likely to burn fat in the future.

If it's important to you to condition your body to go the distance, stimulate your aerobic fat-burning muscle fibers. Anaerobic fast-twitch, sugar-burning muscle fibers cannot sustain you over the long run. Slow-twitch, fat-burning muscle fibers are singularly better suited to face up to the challenges of long-distance living.

Myth
You must burn up your sugar stores
before your body is able to burn fat.

Reality
Your body can burn fat right from
the start of your workout.

The myth that you must first deplete your body of sugar before it can tap into its vast reservoirs of fat is one of the most distracting beliefs of the fitness culture. I overhear this tale being told in locker rooms, and I see it in advertisements and sports journals. The truth is that your body can have immediate access to its fat stores; all you have to do is design the appropriate strategy. In the next section, I will explain in detail how to train your body to get its energy from fat rather than from sugar. For the most part, how you set up your training sessions and what you eat determines where your body gets its energy. If you rush right into a high-intensity workout without doing a slow-and-easy warmup, you will be more likely to burn sugar than fat. Why is this so? Because when you suddenly ask your body to produce a lot of energy, it does so by recruiting anaerobic, fast-twitch muscle fibers that burn sugar. However, if you take your time to get going, your body will rely on its aerobic, slow-twitch muscle fibers that depend on fat as their main energy source.

Also, your body tends to burn what you feed it. If you eat a lot of sugar, your body will tend to burn sugar. Eat a well-balanced diet, and your body will be more likely to burn fat. I will expound on this concept later on in the "How to Eat for the Distance" section. For now, rest assured that burning fat is not necessarily accomplished by pushing your body to the point of sugar exhaustion.

I encourage you to see the big picture and understand that life doesn't have to be either/or. You'll lose the point if you reduce this chapter to the formulation, "Sugar is bad and fat is good." As I explained earlier, sugar-burning serves a critical purpose in our bodies. Your body is always burning low levels of sugar to fuel your nervous system and brain function. The burning of sugar also helps to ignite the burning of fats. Even though we have an almost unlimited availability of fats, we need continual carbohydrate (sugar) metabolism to break them down. Also, while anaerobic muscle fibers are specifically designed to burn sugar, even muscle fibers programmed to burn fat can, in some cases, burn sugar. In the end, it is all a question of balance. Once your body is aerobically healthy and fit, you can benefit from sugar-burning workouts. Until that time, the repeated exposure to sugar-burning training can stress you out and wear you down.

When you're constantly on the go with no time to organize the day properly, it is easy to begin looking for shortcuts. Harder, faster workouts becomes appealing; so does not exercising at all. Eating on the run develops into the norm. It doesn't take much to compromise your commitment to wellness with the rationalization that once your life gets back on track, you'll embrace healthier habits. In the meantime, the lure of high-carbohydrate, sugar-rich foods are all around you, and you indulge because they provide such an immediate and perceptible blast of energy. A temporary solution becomes a habit—and an unsavory recipe for turning your body into a sugar-burning, acid-forming, and fat-storing machine.

A lifestyle ridden with stress, poor training, and unbalanced nutritional practices can lead to a gradual and growing dependency on sugar-based energy production. Once this happens, you will adversely affect your energy level, your mood, and the way your body feels. You will also set in motion a vicious circle of sugar craving and continued sugar-burning (and fat storing) that can gather momentum like a tightly packed snowball rolling down a steep hill covered with wet snow. Your body will not be set up for success in the long run, and your ability to stay healthy and free of illness and disease will be severely jeopardized—not a great way to embark on the long-distance journey of your life.

Soon, I'm going to ask you to consider training and eating in ways that are probably new to you. Before I do, I need to give you compelling reasons to change behavior that has probably been in place for years. I could just say, "Run slower and eat less sugar. It works!" But instead let me describe in detail the hallmarks of sugar-based energy.

SUGAR-BASED ENERGY IS INCONSISTENT

Training or eating to burn sugar can get you through the moment, but what about later? Chances are you'll seriously strain your body's ability to maintain its blood-sugar levels. Once the blood-sugar level become unstable, you are susceptible to frequent energy highs and lows. You impair your mental alertness and ability to focus for long periods.

Have you ever gone out for a long run and reached the point where you couldn't go on? Maybe you experienced this as a sudden drop in your energy level. I have seen and experienced this (when I could have made better choices, of course!) during my competitive racing career and in my coaching practice.

Maybe your experience has been less dramatic. You feel generally irritable and have mercurial moods. Emotional "highs" and "lows" are another symptom of fluctuating blood-sugar levels. Whichever the case, avoid blood-sugar lows if you are committed to continuing on a long-term journey. The best way to elude this de-energizing and debilitating state is to get your body to burn fat, not sugar.

SUGAR-BASED ENERGY MAKES YOU ACIDIC

Ask anyone who's run a marathon about lactic acid and you'll hear day-after tales of having to walk down the stairs backward or about quads that throbbed with pain. Beware. These symptoms are often accompanied by melancholy moods. What's the culprit of both symptoms? Too much lactic acid.

Lactic acid is actually an omnipresent aspect of your body's chemical makeup. As small amounts of sugar are being metabolized into energy, lactic acid is constantly being produced. It travels through the bloodstream to the liver, where it gets converted into sugar (glucose) for use as energy. There is a natural give-and-take to this process in the body. The anaerobic sugar-burning energy system produces the lactic acid, and the aerobic fat-burning system gets rid of it (remember, some sugar-burning is going on in the aerobic fat-burning muscles). The more developed your aerobic fat-burning system is, the more likely it is that you will be able to counterbalance and neutralize the lactic-acid-producing effect of burning sugar. As long as lactic-acid production remains low and manageable, your body can function and flourish.

However, high levels of lactic acid production can inhibit the functioning of the aerobic fat-burning system and produce muscular injury, nervous system irritation (decrease in coordination and motor skills), and, in the most extreme cases, anxiety, depression, and phobias.

Lactic-acid buildup is often caused by a faulty metabolism in which excessive acid is produced and the pH of the blood and tissue is affected. It can also be a result of exercising too intensively, having too much sugar in your diet, and stress. These sugar-burning, acid-forming training regimes, nutritional strategies, and lifestyle practices produce an internal environment that can adversely affect your mood and emotions. Excessive production and accumulation of lactic acid in the body can turn a motivated, positive, excited, and eager outlook on life into one of negativism, anxiety, despair and hopelessness.

In his book *In Fitness and In Health*, Phil Maffetone relates the story of a national-class runner who maintained a fierce training schedule based on anaerobic workouts. During one race in which she was leading, she ran off-course and proceeded to jump off a bridge, a misfortune that crippled her for life. Whether the act was intentional or accidental was never quite known. Maffetone attributed her extreme behavior to the high levels of lactic acid that had been produced during years of high-intensity, sugar-burning exercise training. I have seen fellow competitors, colleagues, clients, and even friends succumb to the devastating effects of emotional exhaustion and psychological burnout. In most instances, backing off and adopting a healthy and balanced nutritional plan and implementing training strategies geared to burning fat can put you back in a positive state.

SUGAR-BASED ENERGY CAUSES PHYSICAL ACHES AND PAINS

Constant and repetitive bouts of sugar-burning stress can be exhausting to your adrenal glands—the body's primary defense mechanisms in the battle against stress and fluctuating blood-sugar levels. The adrenals keep your body energized, satiated with water and electrolytes, and able to handle most routine aches associated with physical duress. However, constant sugar-burning and sugar-eating can exhaust the adrenals and trigger a weakening in the muscle groups with which they are associated. Exhausted and dysfunctional adrenal glands can be related to joint discomfort; fatigue; physical and mental exhaustion; knee, back, and foot problems; and even immune-system disorders. Dysfunctional adrenal glands can also inhibit the secretion of cortisone, the body's natural anti-inflammatory medication. Without the cortisone, mild and natural inflammations resulting from physical training cannot be managed and controlled and can develop into major bodily aches and pains. By turning your body into a sugar burner, you compromise your adrenal health and undermine your ability to remain energized, functioning, and free of muscular discomfort and joint pain.

SUGAR-BASED ENERGY LEADS TO SUGAR CRAVINGS

Think about this: when you run fast for forty-five to sixty minutes, you can burn up about five hundred calories of sugar—nearly 20 percent of your body's total sugar stores. With such a major drop in its emergency and nervous-system fuel stores, your body sends a message to the brain along the lines of, "Get me more sugar!" Imagine the challenge to an endurance person who needs to move for hours—even days—and burn thousands upon thousands of calories. Your body cannot allow its sugar stores (remember, it contains only about 2,500 calories to begin with) to be reduced by more than 25 percent, so it sends out messages to acquire new sources of sugar to replenish what is being drawn out.

On the other hand, since fat stores are nearly unlimited (a minimum of 130,000 calories for most individuals), the loss of even 1,500 calories amounts to a less than a 1-percent reduction in the fuel available in the body's fat-storage warehouse. Your body won't miss them at all. Unlike the case where you use up 1,500 calories of sugar, you won't get urgent messages to go out and replace the used fat.

Burning sugar can lead to excessive carbohydrate ingestion, which in turn can set off a cycle of carbohydrate intolerance, insulin overproduction, and reduced fat metabolism. The impact of insulin on sugar usage and fat storage can be dramatic. In the nutrition section of the book, we will explore in greater detail the role insulin plays in the saga of sugar versus fats. For now it is important to understand that as insulin levels rise, blood sugar levels fall. This up-and-down, rise-and-fall dynamic between insulin and blood sugar is delicate and precise, and throwing it off by the excessive consumption of carbohydrates and sugar-based foods can dramatically affect energy and performance levels.

BURNING SUGAR MAKES YOU VULNERABLE TO COLDS, FLUS, AND ALLERGIES

If you are committed to go the distance and to live life to the fullest, you need to stay healthy. Your best defense against colds, flus, and allergies is to build a strong immune system. The immune system is composed of a complex network of organs containing cells that recognize foreign substances in the body and try to destroy them. It protects the body from such invaders as germs, viruses, and bacteria. When functioning optimally, the immune system can ward off illness and disease. How strong is your immune system? The answer is determined by how well you stave off colds and flus. I notice how often professional athletes are sidelined by cold ailments. It's amazing how many people preparing for a big event get sick right before. What's the correlation? Constant exposure to high-intensity exercise and stress has a disruptive effect on your body's ability to stay healthy and injury-free.

A word to people who want to feel youthful as they age: high-intensity physical activity seems to produces large amounts of free radicals, by-products of energy production that can speed up the aging process. Dr. Thomas Crais, an antiaging expert based in New Orleans, calls these free radicals "little oxidizers of the cells." In effect they cause our cell membranes to rust, just as an old piece of metal would when its scratched surface is exposed to moisture. Under normal conditions these dangerous free radicals can be controlled by the natural antioxidants contained in our body and food. The most well-known antioxidants include vitamins A, C, and E, selenium, beta-carotene, bioflavonoids, taurine, the phenols found in red wine, and enzymes found in the mitochondria, the fat-burning ovens of the muscle cells.

However, regular bouts of high-intensity sugar-burning activity can produce excessive and dangerous levels of free radicals in the body. It can also inhibit the production of health-promoting natural killer cells and stimulate the secretion of cortisol by the adrenal glands. Cortisol, while responsible for helping your body deal with stress, is also an immune-system suppressant. In fact, heart surgeons inject transplant patients with cortisol in order to suppress the patient's immune system so the transplanted organ won't be rejected. For me, the conclusion seems obvious. If you want to be healthy, burn more fat and less sugar.

BURNING SUGAR REDUCES THE AMOUNT OF FAT YOUR BODY BURNS

The more sugar your body burns, the less fat it uses. The less fat your body uses, the less likely you will be able to go the distance. What are the benefits of burning fat? Fat is far more abundant than sugar. Stored fat accounts for more than 80 percent of the calories available as fuel to your body. Fat is stored fuel, your body's most abundant natural resource. Its energy potential is nearly limitless. There is a liberating quality to this physiological fact, and a special place for fat in our heritage. Covert Bailey said it best in his book *Fit or Fat*: when living organisms began storing fat, they liberated themselves from their immediate environment because they were no longer dependent on whatever nutrients surrounded them. The emergence of stored fat was both the extra fuel tank and the new-age fuel that created the possibility of long-distance hunting and gathering.

Burning fat promotes health in ways that burning sugar can't. Unlike the higher intensity fight-or-flight sugar metabolism, the more moderate and peaceful fat-burning system does not promote lactic acid buildup, nor does it stimulate the production of harmful amounts of free radicals. At moderate fat-burning levels of intensity, the body seems to produce a greater amount of natural killer cells to help protect it from viral, bacterial, and fungal attack. Burning fat also stimulates the secretion of natural antioxidants in the body to counteract the harmful effects of free-radical oxidation caused by anaerobic stress. And, as sugar-burning seems to beget more sugar-burning, fat-burning begets more fat-burning. How does this process occur? First of all, when you produce energy aerobically, by burning fat, you stimulate the growth in size and number of the mitochondria, the fat-burning "ovens" found in the muscle cells. Secondly, aerobic fat-burning activity increases your sensitivity to insulin. Increased insulin sensitivity means a diminished presence of this sugar-burning, fat-storing hormone, reduces the likelihood of hyper (high) insulin production, and promotes stable blood sugar levels. These factors combine to move your body toward an ever-increasing state of stable and consistent energy output and fat-burning aerobic health.

The more training you do in fat-burning zones, the healthier your blood will be and the calmer, less stressed out you'll feel. Aerobic fat-burning exercise clears the blood of fats after you eat. It also promotes optimal circulation and blood-lipid (fat) profiles by decreasing blood-platelet aggregation (clumping of the blood) and clogging of the arteries. Aerobic fat-burning exercise calms you down by generating the secretion of chemicals that stimulate the parasympathetic nervous system, which tends to have a calming effect on your body.

THE PROS OF FAT BURNING

- Increases the size and number of mitochondria, the fat-burning "ovens" found in the muscles
- Increases insulin sensitivity, reducing the likelihood of hyper (high) insulin production and promoting stable blood-sugar levels and the burning of fat
- Increases the body's ability to clear the blood of triglycerides after eating
- Increases the secretion of chemicals that stimulate the parasympathetic nervous system and foster relaxation
- Promotes optimal circulation and blood-lipid (fat) profiles by decreasing blood-platelet aggregation and clogging of the arteries

In conclusion, the biggest mistake that people make in an endurance-training program is unwittingly and inadvertently training their bodies to rely more on sugar than fat. For staying power, maximum endurance, and optimal health, fat is the fuel of choice. Fat represents the greatest source of energy available to the human body. When your body burns fat it not only taps into a huge reservoir of energy, but it also has a profound and positive impact on the biochemistry of your body, its structure, and, ultimately, your mood and your ability to remain focused and alert for extended periods. Endurance is not only about the quantity of available energy, but also its quality. In effect, we have two fuel tanks. And it is the fat tank that will fuel us to go the distance.

How Well Do You Burn Fat?

A number of methodologies, which vary in accessibility and cost, can measure how much fat your body is able to burn:

- gas-exchange analysis
- blood analysis
- oral pH
- questionnaire

Some tests are simple, and you can do them yourself. Others require special equipment available only at gyms or nearby colleges. Costs range from a few dollars for litmus paper and the oral pH test to hundreds of dollars for a gas-exchange analysis. In my practice, we use variations of all four methods.

GAS-EXCHANGE ANALYSIS

The most effective way to test your fat-burning ability is to do a metabolic performance analysis using a carbon dioxide/oxygen analyzer. Also known as a metabolic cart, the carbon dioxide/oxygen analyzer monitors how much of your energy comes from burning fat and how much from burning sugar. The test itself is called a substrate-utilization analysis. The word *substrate* refers to the amount of a given fuel source—carbohydrates (sugar) or fats—your body uses to produce energy. It is possible to identify the pattern of energy use by monitoring the oxygen and carbon-dioxide content of inspired and expired air.

How the test works:

In an exercise lab the subject works out on a stationary bike or motorized treadmill while breathing into a mouthpiece connected by a tube to an oxygen/carbon dioxide analyzer. By comparing the oxygen and carbon dioxide content of room air to the oxygen and carbon dioxide content of the person's expired air, the carbon dioxide/oxygen analyzer determines how much oxygen is being consumed and how much carbon dioxide is being produced. If the amount of oxygen you consume is greater than the amount of carbon dioxide you produce, you are a good fat burner. If the amount of carbon dioxide you produce is greater than the amount of oxygen consumed, you are a sugar burner. Physiologists term the point at which carbon dioxide production is radically greater than oxygen consumption as the ventilation breakpoint (VB).

The VO2max test is a similar procedure. While it uses a nearly identical data-collection method, the procedures and diagnostic techniques vary. VO2max tests measure a person's aerobic capacity, which refers to the maximum amount of oxygen (in milliliters) your heart, lungs, and blood vessels are capable of delivering to your working muscles per minute per kilogram of body weight. Substrate-utilization analysis uses a similar data-collection technology, but instead of focusing just on oxygen consumed, it is equally interested in the amount of carbon dioxide produced.

When your body burns sugar, it produces more carbon dioxide per unit of oxygen than when it burns fat. You might already be aware of this phenomenon. Earlier I mentioned that the location, sound, and feel of your breathing is an indicator where you're getting your energy from. When you've burning fat, your breathing is quiet, low to the belly, and relaxed. As you begin to move into a greater sugar-burning fight-or-flight intensity, your breathing becomes shallower and more rapid, moves higher up in the chest, and is accompanied by a noticeable forced expulsion of air. This heavier breathing, a conspicuous gasping or panting for air, is part of the body's dynamic of sugar-burning. Burning sugar produces acid, which begins to lower the pH of the blood. Your body neutralizes or buffers the acid, using natural bicarbonates in the blood. The end product of this buffering process is the production of carbon dioxide, which is literally blown out of the body as you exhale. Using a oxygen/carbon dioxide analyzer, we can detect this rise in carbon dioxide production and determine the moment when the shift takes place. Thus, we can determine what is the heart rate range where maximum fat utilization occurs, when sugar usage begins to increase, and finally when all fat-burning cease and sugar becomes the exclusive fuel of choice. With this information, training programs can be designed to emphasize fat utilization, improve energy levels, and maximize endurance.

BLOOD ANALYSIS

The other well known methodology for determining how well you burn fat is to test the lactic-acid concentration of your blood to find your blood-lactate threshold. The blood-lactate threshold represents the point at which blood lactate (lactic acid) is produced at a faster rate than it is removed and begins to accumlate in the blood. This threshold point goes by many names, the most common of which are: The onset of blood lactate accumulation (OBLA) or anaerobic threshold (AT).

Blood-lactate testing is considered the gold standard in determining the point at which the body has turning exclusively anaerobic, sugar-burning, and acidic. However, it doesn't tell you the percent of energy that comes from fat and the percent that comes from sugar. Only the oxygen/carbon dioxide analyzer can do that.

How the test works:

Blood analysis tests are offered at many university research facilities; some at-home versions are beginning to appear. Also, check the Internet for kits and mail-in labs. In all instances, you or an attending health professional take a blood test, which is sent to a lab for analysis.

ORAL pH

A less precise but more accessible and dramatically less costly measurement technique involves the use of litmus paper to measure oral pH. The technique was first introduced by Dr. George Goodheart and has been further refined by his followers, most notably Dr. Philip Maffetone. The test is based on the assumption that the more acidic your mouth becomes (the lower your pH), the more likely it is that sugar is being used as energy. Again, the oral pH testing procedure is based on the logic that burning sugar produces acid, which can manifest itself by lowering the pH of the saliva in the mouth. Conversely, the higher the pH, the more alkaline the mouth, the more likely fat is being used. You can purchase pH paper at many pharmaceutical- or medical-supply stores. I suggest you purchase pH paper with a range of 6.0 to 8.0.

Most often, you can identify your pH by noting the color of the litmus paper after you moisten it with saliva. When a person's saliva is acidic, the paper will appear yellow. The greater the alkalinity of the saliva, the darker the paper gets. As a general rule, the litmus paper will transform from yellow to yellow-green to green to greenish-blue to blue. Each color corresponds to a numerical pH that is identified in the chart that comes with the paper.

How the test works:

The pH of your mouth can be taken simply by breaking off a small piece of the litmus paper and wetting it with the saliva in your mouth. Check with the manufacturer, or read the label to see if the paper can be put directly in your mouth. If it can't, spit in a cup and dip the paper there. The color of the paper will then change in proportion to the degree of acidity in your mouth. Usually, the less the paper color changes, the lower the pH and the greater the acidity. Conversely, when the color of the paper changes noticeably, it is an indication of a higher pH and greater alkalinity in your mouth.

This method is controversial. Other factors can affect the pH of the mouth. For instance, dental problems and tooth decay can lower the pH of the mouth. What you just ate can affect the test, although if you refrain from eating for at least twenty minutes, you will probably not skew the outcome of the test. We do use this testing method when we work with large groups or correspond with clients around the world. We also use the litmus paper technique to monitor specific training sessions. You can test the pH of your mouth at various stages during a workout. Before you start your training session, test the pH of your mouth as described above. Check your pH again during your workout and one more time when you are done. If, for instance, you are scheduled for an aerobic fat-burning training session, the litmus paper will get darker, indicating that your are less acidic at the end of the workout than at the beginning. If this is true, you have reason to be confident that your target-zone settings are working and your nutritional strategies are balanced. On the other hand, if the color of the paper doesn't change or gets lighter as the workout progresses, this would indicate that you are not increasing the amount of fat you are burning or you are burning more sugar and your body is becoming more acidic. Should your body turn more acidic during a training session, it is a signal that you might be exercising too hard (burning sugar produces acid) or your nutritional strategies may be too rich in carbohydrates (sugar). Check with the chart that follows to see where you stand with respect to your fat-metabolizing capability.

yellow	yellow-green	green	greenish-blue	blue

6.0 6.4 6.8 7.0 7.2 7.6 8.0

Poor Fat Metabolizer ———————— Good Fat Metabolizer

Note: Litmus paper comes with a chart that matches the color of the paper with your numerical pH.

Quiz: Are You a Sugar Burner or a Fat Burner?

Answer these questions and total your score to determine your fat-burning ability.

QUESTION 1: ENERGY LEVELS

How often does your energy level fluctuate throughout the day?

1 constantly
2 often
3 sometimes
4 rarely
5 never

QUESTION 2: POSTEXERCISE ENERGY LEVELS

How do you feel after you exercise?

1 always exhausted/never energized
2 often exhausted/rarely energized
3 sometimes exhausted/sometimes energized
4 rarely exhausted/often energized
5 never exhausted/always energized

QUESTION 3: POSTEXERCISE BODY FEELINGS

When you exercise, how often do you experience bodily aches and pains, especially in your knees or lower back?

1 constantly
2 often
3 sometimes
4 rarely
5 never

QUESTION 4: FOOD-CRAVING TENDENCIES

How often do you find yourself craving carbohydrates or something sweet to eat?
1 constantly
2 often
3 sometimes
4 rarely
5 never

QUESTION 5: FOOD-AVOIDANCE TENDENCIES

How often do you make an effort to eat only those foods or food products labeled as fat-free, low-fat, or nonfat?
1 constantly
2 often
3 sometimes
4 rarely
5 never

QUESTION 6: IMMUNE-SYSTEM FUNCTION

How often do you experience colds, flus, or allergy symptoms?
1 constantly
2 often
3 sometimes
4 rarely
5 never

Your Total Score	Fat-Burning Ability
5–12	Poor
13–21	Fair
22–30	Good

QUESTIONNAIRE ANALYSIS

Energy levels:

If your energy level fluctuates constantly throughout the day, you are probably prone to burning sugar, not fat. Using carbohydrates and blood sugar as the main energy source for aerobic muscular activity (instead of fat) can lead to mood swings and physical and mental fatigue.

Postexercise energy and feelings:

If you often feel weary and exhausted after working out, you are either working out too hard or not burning fat. Exercising at intensities above your target heart rate reduces the amount of fat you burn and forces you to use stored carbohydrates—muscle glycogen and blood sugar—for energy.

Improper warm-up techniques, rapid increases in heart rate, and constant fluctuations in heart rate during your workout also limit the amount of fat your body uses for energy.

Food-craving tendencies:

If you are usually hungry in the morning or after working out, you may not be eating enough high-quality essential fatty oils. Without ingestion of some dietary fat, your body will be less likely to use stored body fat for energy and will be more likely to use stored carbohydrates during exercise and at rest.

Immune-system function:

Your best defense against colds, flus, and allergies is to build a strong immune system. The immune system is composed of a complex network of organs containing cells that recognize foreign substances in the body and try to destroy them. It protects the body from invaders such as germs, viruses, and bacteria. When functioning optimally, the immune system can ward off illness and disease. The strength of your immune system is determined by whether you get enough of the right exercise, what kinds of foods you eat, how well you manage stress, and how much you rely on sugar as an energy source.

15

Structure Leads to Freedom

Now that you that know burning fat is the key to effortless endurance, how can you train your body to burn more fat? Simple—just figure out when you're burning fat and design a training program based upon heart-rate monitoring that will take you there more often. Before I tell you how to put together a heart-rate monitoring training program, I will share with you how I got involved with this technology in the first place. My original infatuation with heart-rate monitors and target-zone strategies stemmed from a desire to understand what was happening to me as I trained. I wanted more than to simply go out every day and do whatever I felt like. Early on I had no plan other than to run as much and for as long as I could. On certain days I'd run harder than on others—when I felt like it. On other days I'd take it easy, if that was all I wanted to do. Yet too many times I wondered if I was wasting my time. Was I getting anywhere? I fell into the trap of measuring and assessing my progress in terms of how well I performed each and every day. That became a painful and disconcerting path, turning into a cycle of trying to outdo myself each time I went out, either for training runs or competitive events.

I wanted to enjoy running and feel as though I was benefiting physically, emotionally, and intellectually. Later on, as a coach, I wanted to draw from the experiences I had to make my life and the lives of others better. I wanted it all, enjoyment of the process and a sense of what Tony Robbins likes to call "Constant and Never-Ending Improvement" (CANI). What I needed was a lodestar, a guiding principle that could help me organize my thoughts in an effective way. I wanted to go beyond just saying to someone, "Listen to your body" or "Run based on how you feel" when too often the person had no idea what to "look," "listen," or "feel" for.

I view physical training, the process of physical mastery, as an apprenticeship, similar to learning how to play a musical instrument. From the onset, you have to commit yourself to learning the tools of the trade. The most accomplished musician must first learn from a master the proper way to hold the instrument, practice playing the scales until they become second nature, and perhaps learn how to read notes on sheets of music. The objective isn't to hold the instrument, play the scales, and read the music. The ultimate goal is to be free of these concerns and just play. You want to be creative, feel at one with the instrument, and make music, not just repeat scales. Until the music student goes through this process, the command to go out and play music may make no sense whatsoever.

Let your heart-rate monitor and target-zone schedule be your scales and sheet music. The goal isn't to follow the schedule. The goal is to draw out your physical talent and empower yourself to compose your own symphony. The heart-rate monitor and training schedule are simply tools for you and your "master" or coach to convey information and assess progress. Each workout is like playing a different scale, creating and surmounting a new challenge. When the time comes to "play," your creativity will emerge because you took the time to practice your scales. This is why you learn to use a heart-rate monitor so that you can perform without one.

The point is not to force your body to do that which it does not want. Having a schedule simply means having a plan. Once you design a plan, you can change the plan if it doesn't seem to fit or if it's no longer working. Much of my coaching takes place over the phone or via e-mail or fax and involves fine-tuning the initial target zones based upon the experience my client is having. We can do this because we have a blueprint, a structure, a concrete plan that we both refer to as a basis for communicating our ideas and suggestions about how to proceed. Without this common language of target zones, we'd be challenged to transfer information and express our thoughts.

As I've done with my clients, I want to encourage you to figure out your target heart-rate zones and create an individualized training program. As you train in your target heart-rate zones, your focus will shift from how hard you can push yourself to how productive you can be while remaining in the prescribed target heart-rate zones. In other words, you will no longer be given the assignment of running at a certain pace for a specific amount of time. I am offering a different kind of challenge: to move within a certain zone, defined by a target heart rate, for a given duration. For a lot of people, this assignment is a radical departure from conventional training. Ask most any runner how a training session went, and he or she will answer along the lines of, "I ran three miles at a seven-minute-thirty-second-mile pace." Or "I ran faster or slower today than yesterday." Most runners assess how well they did by how fast they ran. But the more empowering perspective isn't about speed, it's about how productive you can be while remaining in a relatively comfortable and aerobic fat-burning state. If the only way to be productive and fast is to move into a more urgent anaerobic sugar-burning state, then you're missing the point! Heart-rate monitoring techniques will challenge you to rely more on the experience your body is having than on how fast you can make yourself move. Are you in a comfortable aerobic state using fat as energy, in a more urgent anaerobic state in which your only fuel is sugar, or somewhere in between? The way to distinguish these states is how the world looks, sounds, feels, smells, and tastes as you move. Your body experiences this composite of sights, sounds, feelings, flavors, and aromas. It doesn't know the rate at which it moves.

When we focus on speed, we take ourselves out of our bodies. The body can't comprehend minutes per mile and kilometers. These measurements are just an arbitrary construct, an abstraction of sorts, that is the product of the mind. In nature, there are no miles, nor is pace something that intuitively makes sense to the body. These concepts are figments of your mental processing.

Using a monitor, your focus will shift from miles and pace to how well you can keep your heart rate in a prescribed target zone. You can train yourself to become more aware and connected to the experience your body is having. What your mind thinks of as fast or slow, your body experiences as the sights, sounds, and feelings of the world around you and the myriad thoughts and emotions that run through your mind: the range of colors in the landscape, the shape of the cloud formations spread out in the sky, the sound of birds chirping and the wind blowing, or the feel of your feet making contact with the ground.

If you're extending yourself, your body knows it's running fast not by your watch but by the blurring of the scenery into a two-dimensional "tunnel" as your attention is drawn to a spot in front of you. Your hearing will be overwhelmed by the sound of the forced expulsion of air as you kick the effort level up a notch. Depending on your pace, you will either feel comfortable or tense, relaxed or alarmed.

Most people are not tuned in to this level of sensory-based information as they exercise. We are so conditioned to focus on results rather than the quality of our experience. By determining your target heart rate and training in specific zones, you can be in touch with your body and the information it provides. Then and only then can you make empowering decisions about what is best to do. You can run to seek an at-oneness with your body. You can run to be comfortable and confident about your physicality and how you look. You can run to have the energy to do all the things you want to do.

It is 1994, and I am in Hawaii training a new client, Paul. I barely get my first sentence out when Paul declares to me, "I am not a runner. The only reason I'm here is that I want more energy." He explains that he's never been athletic, but as a real-estate developer with long hours, he needs an exercise program for endurance and energy that doesn't leave him burnt out and exhausted.

I strap a heart-rate monitor around his chest and off we run. After several minutes, I determine his comfortable, aerobic state, set his target zone, and talk him through the sensory markers of this fat-burning world: he hears the waves and birds, sees the beach and sunbathers, feels the warmth of the sun. We run easily in this state for about forty-five minutes. When we stop, I tell Paul we've run four-and-a-half miles. He replies, "I didn't have a good workout. I'm not exhausted." I explain that if endurance and energy are his goals, he needs to train in this comfortable fat-burning state. I design a training program based on his heart rate, and he promises to come back in a year. Paul has come back to train with me each year for the past four years. I've seen him transformed from a man who hated exercise to someone who can't live without it. He runs in his target heart-rate zones for one hour every day. This amazes me, coming from a man whose first words were, "I'm not a runner." He continues to look forward to this daily ritual; it's his anchor. He tells me, "I do this because I love feeling great."

Like Paul, at the start of your new program, training in your target zone may feel so much easier than you're accustomed to that you wonder, what's the point? All I ask is that you wait before you abandon the plan. For many, creating an aerobic fat-burning ballast to an anaerobically excessive life is absolutely the first order of business. This may require repetitive training experiences unlike anything you've had in the past. You may have to hold back to train your body to use more fat as fuel. The objective, however, isn't to stay calm and peaceful forever. No way! The objective is to have it all, calm and relaxing, efficient and productive, stimulating and up-tempo. I want your life to be filled with unbounded energy, optimal health, unrelenting happiness, and total fulfill-ment. I want you to be able to go farther, go longer, and go beyond every boundary and limitation you ever imagined. I want your physical destiny to be filled with joy and awe. I want you to be amazed at the possibilities. It can start with such humble beginnings, like the first step of a thousand-mile race, and end with an outcome you that you could have foreseen only in your wildest dreams.

So, yes, you may start off exercising in a zone that seems too easy. Through time, though, thanks to feedback from the heart-rate monitor and the training schedule you will soon create, your capacity to perform and your ability to get things accomplished will improve spectacularly while you remain in a relatively com-fortable state. You will get more done without having to work harder. Incredible! And once your mind, body, and diet are in sync and your fat-burning ability is high, up-tempo challenges will no longer debilitate you and break you down. Once you learn to appreciate and master being calm and moving slowly, you will enjoy being forceful and going hard when the occasions arise. That is the possibility and my promise to you.

16

Stu's Recipe for Heart-Rate Zones

Now you're ready to figure out your target heart-rate zones and create a personalized training program for unmistakable and lasting progress. A target heart-rate zone can guide you to your most effective energy-producing state. The zone itself is just a number, a range of possible heart rates defined by an upper or lower limit in which you will move on any day. The zone itself can be set for anything. The range can be set to keep you relaxed, comfortable, aerobic, and fat-burning or move you into a more demanding, urgent, anaerobic, sugar-burning mode. The range can also be somewhere in between, a space that feels productive and efficient yet free of pressure and alarm.

My training system is organized around these three possible heart-rate ranges that I call cardio c-quences. Your mostly aerobic pace, or the MAP cardio c-quence, is the most comfortable zone in which to train. In the MAP zone, you are aerobic and fat-burning. On the other end is the speedy anaerobic pace or the SAP cardio c-quence. In this zone you feel noticeably challenged, in a state of greater stress and strain, with a sense of urgency and alarm. During these times you enter the anaerobic world of sugar-burning. In between is a narrow middle zone that I call the most efficient pace or the MEP cardio c-quence. In this precise, precariously situated zone, you have the heightened awareness of a tightrope walker. You must be completely focused on the moment, in the present. You must not daydream for a second or fantasize about the future or you might lose your balance and fall out of the zone. The MEP, the most productive and efficient mixed-fuel zone, occupies the space between the fat-burning and sugar-burning extremes. In truth, there could be a fourth zone that is a frenzied, explosive, and a flee-because-your-life-is-in-danger-intensity sprint. I rarely train in this zone intentionally, and I certainly don't encourage many of my clients to. For the average athlete who is not engaged in professional competition, the risks of getting into this furious all-out alarm mode far outweigh the benefits. Repeated exposure to this extreme intensity does little to prepare you for an event of marathon proportions. You're never going to be at this all-out state during the event. When and if the time comes to fight for your survival, the well-trained athlete can draw upon strengths he or she never imagined possible.

Many different formulas and methodologies can predict your heart-rate zones. The gas-exchange and blood-lactate analysis methodologies described in chapter 14 identify the point at which the body transforms from being an aerobic fat-burning machine into an all-out sugar burner. In response to the growing demand for these tests, some health clubs have begun to offer them, but they remain costly and hard to find. By far the greatest number of people base their heart-rate programs on target zones derived from one of several mathematical formulas. These formulas can be useful—indeed, I relied on them when I first started training with a heart-rate monitor. Now I find them less precise than I would like and, for reasons that I will identify below, not as empowering as they could be. Still, just so you understand the context within which my formula emerged—and so you'll understand the formulas when other people bring them up—I will briefly review the two most common target heart-rate zone setting formulas.

The most well known mathematical equation establishes a target range by taking a percentage of your predicted (or actual) maximum heart rate (HRmax). To calculate your predicted maximum heart rate, subtract your age from 220. Your target training zone lies between 70 and 85 percent of the number that represents your predicted HRmax. To calculate this range, simply multiply your predicted maximum heart rate by .70 to establish the lower limit and .85 to establish the upper limit. For example, here's the formula for the target heart-rate zone for a forty-eight-year-old:

The upper limit: 220 − 48 or 172 × (.85) or 146 The lower limit: 220 − 48 or 172 × (.70), or 120. Thus, according to the HRmax formula, the recommended training zone for a person who is forty-eight years of age is between 120 and 146.

Another popular mathematical formula is the heart-rate reserve (HRR), or Karvonen formula. This equation further personalizes the HRmax formula by taking into account your resting pulse (RP). While there is a wide variance in the resting pulse in the general population, most people have a resting pulse between sixty and eighty beats per minute (bpm). I've worked with untrained or aerobically unfit individuals with resting pulses as high as ninety to a hundred bpm and with aerobically fit and endurance-trained athletes having resting pulses as low as forty to fifty bpm. My resting pulse, for instance, is usually in the low to mid forties. These differences can affect the setting of your optimal target heart-rate zones. Take two people of the same age, for instance, one with a resting pulse of forty-four, the other with a resting pulse of seventy-five. Setting a target training zone based solely on each person's age might not accurately reflect these basic physiological differences. To address this, the Karvonen formula takes into account your resting pulse in determining your target zone. The key is first establishing the heart-rate reserve. The heart-rate reserve is, simply and logically, the range between your resting pulse and predicted maximum heart rate. To identify your heart-rate reserve, subtract your resting pulse from your predicted maximum heart rate, or 220 minus your age minus your resting pulse. The range is now compressed, because the lower limit is your resting pulse, not zero, as was the case when using the HRmax formula. Hence, when using the HRR equation, the percentages shift downward to 60 to 80 percent instead of the 70 to 85 percent limits of the HRmax. (Once you calculate the percentage range, you'll need to add the resting pulse back in to the calculation.) Thus, for me—and using forty-four bpm as my resting pulse—my training zone, according to HRR logic is as follows:

For the upper limit: (220 − age − resting pulse × .80) + resting pulse

$$(220 - 48 - 44) \times (.80) + 44$$
$$(128 \times .80) + 44$$
$$102.4 + 44 = 146$$

For the lower limit: (220 − age − resting pulse × .60) + resting pulse

$$(220 - 48 - 44) \times (.60) + 44$$
$$(128 \times .60) + 44$$
$$76.8 + 44 = 120.8 \text{ or } 121$$

As you can see, in this case both the HRmax and the HRR predict almost the identical target zone range: 120 (or 121) to 146. This is not always the case however, especially if your resting pulse is particularly high.

As I mentioned earlier, you can use either the HRmax or HRR to guide you in your training. Keep your heart rate toward the lower end and you'll burn more fat; at the upper end you'll burn more sugar. However, I do have specific challenges with these equations:

• The zones are wide and "all-encompassing." The experience of exercising at the lower end of the zone can be very different from the upper end. For most people the lower ends of the zone calculated by these methods are comfortable, fat-burning, and aerobic, while the upper ends elicit the more intense, sugar-burning, and anaerobic experience. Just putting yourself "anywhere" in the zone doesn't help you distinguish when you're burning fat or sugar.

• A single target zone doesn't distinguish the range of experiences you have when you move. Most people are in one of three "states" when they move: comfortable and relaxed, working hard and straining, or somewhere in between—a place I call efficient and productive. To reflect these three experiences, my training system relies on the three heart-rate ranges (cardio c-quences) mentioned earlier: the comfortable, aerobic, and fat-burning MAP (mostly aerobic pace); the efficient and productive mixed-fuel MEP (most efficient pace); and, finally, the anaerobic, challenging, and sugar-burning SAP (speedy anaerobic pace). Neither the HRmax nor the HRR formula is that helpful in distinguishing these zones.

• Wide zones don't allow you to effectively monitor your training progress. Relying on a wide target zone containing a variety of experiences hinders your ability to notice progress. To effectively track progress and monitor results, a narrower zone is preferable. By concentrating on a smaller heart-rate range and limiting the experience to a more precisely defined and stable state, you are in a better position to evaluate the effectiveness of your training program and to assess the impact it has on your ability to produce results.

Find Your Target Heart-Rate Zones: Five Easy Steps

My recipe for setting target heart rates uses a straightforward and simple formula as a launching point to identify all three possible training zones. It borrows from the work of Dr. Phil Maffetone, a pioneer in the field of heart-rate monitoring. Maffetone recommends subtracting your age from 180 to calculate the upper limit of your target zone. Subtract ten from that number and you have a ten-beat range within which to move. To account for individual differences, he adjusts the entire zone up or down in five-to-ten beat increments. The zone moves up by five to ten beats (see the chart on Stu's recipe for heart-rate zones that follows) for healthy, well-trained endurance athletes, drops by five beats for those just starting out, and is lowered by ten beats for anyone on medication or recovering from a recent illness. For everyone else it stays the same.

A well-trained forty-eight-year-old athlete like me would calculate the upper limit to a 10-beat zone as follows: $180 - 48 = 132$. The 10-beat target-training zone becomes 122 to 132. Because I am an endurance athlete, I adjust the zone up by 10 beats for a target-training zone of 132 to 142. Maffetone's equation produces a narrow 10-beat target training zone that reflects what I call the MEP. The MEP is ideal for monitoring changes and is a fairly accurate way to distinguish the comfortable aerobic and fat-burning movement experience from the more challenging aerobic and stressful sugar-burning one. Above the MEP lies the SAP, where energy production would be considered anaerobic and sugar-burning; below the MEP resides the MAP, where movement is predominately aerobic and fat-burning. While I retain the narrow 10-beat range of the MEP, I recommend that the MAP and SAP be extended to 20 beats. Thus, to formulate the MAP, the lower limit of the MEP is extended downward 20 beats to a range of 112 to 132. The SAP is extended 20 beats upward from the upper limit of the MEP, creating a range of 142 to 162. Thus, beginning with Maffetone's simple (180 minus your age) equation, you can formulate all three of your possible cardio c-quences in a matter of seconds:

Recipe for Stu's Heart-Rate Zones

1. Determine the MEP upper limit: 180 minus your age   *133 + 5 = 138*

   MEP upper limit

2. Determine the MEP lower limit: MEP upper limit minus 10   *123 + 5 = 128*

   MEP lower limit

3. Adjust the MEP zone only if you fall into one of the following categories:

   a. Raise the MEP zone by 10 beats if you are an experienced endurance athlete (three or more hours of aerobic activity per week).

   b. Raise the MEP zone by 5 beats if you are currently engaged in a regular exercise program, but not necessarily endurance trained (fewer than three hours of aerobic activity per week).

   c. Lower the MEP zone by 5 beats if you are just starting out.

   d. Lower the MEP zone by 10 beats if you are on medication or recovering from a recent illness.

   If you do not fall into categories a, b, c, or d, keep the MEP zone as originally calculated. Write your final MEP target zone lower and upper limits in the space below.

   _____   —   _____
   MEP lower limit   MEP upper limit

4. Calculate the lower limit of your MAP by subtracting 20 from the lower limit of the MEP:

   Lower limit of MEP minus 20 = _____

5. Calculate the upper limit of your SAP by adding 20 to the upper limit of the MEP:

   Upper limit of MEP plus 20 = _____

   _____ = (–) 20 _____ – _____ + 20 = _____
   MAP lower limit   MEP lower limit   MEP upper limit   SAP upper limit
                          (MAP upper limit)   (SAP lower Limit)

6. Write your final cardio c-quences below:

   MAP   _____ to _____

   MEP   _____ to _____

   SAP   _____ to _____

Fine-Tuning the Target Zones

Before we move on, I want to emphasize one point: no single formula is right for everyone. Take me, for instance. As I pointed out earlier, traditional heart-rate formulas predict my target workout zone between 120 and 146. Yet I do the bulk of my running between 100 and 125. If I were to train near 146, it'd be tough. I could do it, but I would neither want to nor enjoy training there every day. I have learned to adjust my target zones upward or downward because I know what each zone looks, sounds, and feels like. I can't imagine I would have continued to run as much and as often as I do if I had to force myself to stay in the target zones that traditional formulas recommend.

Imagine, however, if a beginning runner calculated his zones according to the traditional formulas and felt miserable while training in them. Unless he is confident about his body, he might not follow his intuition and make the necessary adjustments for the target zones to work better. It can work the other way also. The formulas can also predict zones that are too low. I have new clients who want to give up on using the heart-rate monitor because the training is so understimulating that it's not worth getting off the couch for.

What I teach my clients and what I would like to share with you is this: the formulas don't know the state you are in. Only you can know. A formula can't tell whether you are aerobic and fat-burning or anaerobic and sugar-burning. Formulas are just best guesses based on the general tendencies of the population at large. While they relate to the world in general, they may pertain to no one in particular. Don't become a prisoner of the numbers. Your goal is to have a training experience that puts you in the energy-producing state prescribed for that day, whether it is aerobic fat-burning, anaerobic sugar-burning, or the mixed-fuel transition zone. Don't stick with a training experience that doesn't make sense to you and your body just because a formula told you so. No one formula is right for everyone.

Bringing the Zones to Life

Now that you have completed the initial calculations and derived all the relevant numbers, I want you to become familiar with the sights, sounds, and feelings that are distinct to each cardio c-quence. Once you are able to access the zones in terms of what they look, sound, and feel like, you will be one step—indeed, one giant step—closer to mastering your physical destiny.

YOUR MOSTLY AEROBIC PACE (MAP)

This target zone is relatively peaceful. It promotes fat utilization, health, and getting to know your body. The percentage of total energy production that comes from fat is at its highest relative levels in the MAP, but since the stimulation is relatively low, you are not burning up a huge amount of calories. You are in the MAP and burning fat when you go out for a long walk, easy jog, or—if you are a more experienced athlete—perform recovery runs after a competition. Feeling comfortable and releasing tension and stress are the key elements of your MAP experience. You want your MAP sessions to be free of anxiety and pressure. Your goal is to move for the sake of moving. Use your time in the MAP to burn fat, to get to know your body, and to inventory the relative degree of tension and relaxation in it as you move toward a deeper state of calm and fluidity.

Visual anchors:

Look for the depth and dimensionality of the world. Note the textures and colors around you. Visual information is expansive; you are able to see things across a wide expanse of vision, both straight ahead and peripherally. You can observe the sky above, the other runners moving about you, or even notice what they are wearing and the way they move. Not only does the map zone allow you access to an exquisite level of detail when viewing the external visual world, it affords you an opportunity to access your internal world as well. You can imagine yourself in your past, maybe the last time you were running on a beach or your last race experience. The images can come to life as you continue moving, uninterrupted by the daydreaming going on in your head. You can see the future. Imagine what it would be like to run in a marathon, see an old friend, or maybe even get a good night's sleep. You can freely associate with anything you want without affecting your ability to move forward.

Auditory anchors:

In your MAP zone, there is a crystalline quality to the sounds around you, as though they are suspended all about you with silent spaces in between, waiting for your radar to pick them up. Your breathing is quiet and unobtrusive, opening the floodgate for a stream of sounds that continually swirl around you. Often, I challenge clients to pick out as many different sounds as possible—birds chirping, waves crashing against the shore, or horns honking—while moving in the MAP.

Kinesthetic anchors:

Again, relaxed and flowing are the keywords for this zone. You experience a profound sense of being at one with the world around you. You are part of nature and the natural flow of life. You are not running past or away from the objects that surround you; they seem to be floating in toward you. Time unfolds according to its own plan. There is nothing to do but flow, become the motion, and let your experience happen. The opportunity exists for you to get to know who you are and what is gong on inside of you that day, emotionally, physically, and spiritually. The MAP exists because you need this time to be yourself. You are not getting anywhere while you are in it. You are creating the possibility that you can be who you are and learn to be comfortable with yourself and your body. Open up your senses and take it all in.

Ask yourself what is the experience you are having right here, right now. What is it you see, what is it you hear, what is it you feel. It is all there for the taking. Seize it; be it!

RPE index:

The rate of perceived exertion (RPE) index can be used to rate your effort level on a scale of zero to ten, where zero is the absolute easiest you can imagine working and ten is the absolute hardest. Your MAP sessions can be anywhere between three and five, depending on your health and fitness level.

Breathing:

Your breath is noticeably quiet, low to the belly, and void of the hyperventilation and forced expulsion of air that typically accompanies exercising at higher sugar-burning intensities.

Energy levels:

Because of its reliance on fat-based energy production, the MAP zone promotes stable and calm energy levels. No matter what your energy level is going into a MAP, when you are done, you will feel better; have more energy, and be more in touch with yourself. For me this remains one of the most appealing aspects of the MAP. I am convinced that moving in the MAP generates energy. When I am tired or feeling low, the MAP is where I head. That is where I go when I want more energy. No matter how down my energy level is, no matter how sluggish or tired I feel, once I perform my MAP, I am in a better place. The MAP is rejuvenating and refreshing. When I am in it, I am reminded how good it feels to be alive and moving forward. I make every attempt possible to schedule my MAP sessions in the morning. It leaves me feeling calm, excited, peaceful, and energized.

Your Most Efficient Pace (MEP)

The MEP, or most efficient pace, is a transition state that straddles the MAP and SAP. This zone represents your most productive and efficient pace. It offers a fabulous balance of productivity and comfort; it provides a maximal return from a minimal effort. In the MEP you feel in control and composed—"within yourself," as athletes like to say—not overextended or on the verge of it. You are in touch with your body and the world around you. You are cognizant of being productive and relatively comfortable at the same time; enlivened with the spirit of confidence that you can continue moving in a state that you can manage and control, and for which you can maintain a sense of mastery. This middle zone—the MEP—is a special place to train; it strikes a balance between the calming peaceful aerobic, fat-burning state and the urgent fast-paced anaerobic sugar-burning world (SAP). Thus, once you find your middle zone, all three cardio c-quences (MAP, MEP, and SAP) become immediately apparent.

The MEP must be sustainable, but not as effortless as the MAP. When it comes to performance enhancement, the MEP is the most significant of the cardio c-quences. When you want to accomplish something, you go there. The MEP is the cardio c-quence you want to be in when you are performing for an extended period and getting results is key. This is especially true for an endurance type of test such as a marathon. The productivity you have in your MEP is the best predictor of your marathon time. Whatever pace (minutes per mile, or miles per hour) you are able to sustain while keeping your heart rate within the boundaries of the MEP, upper and lower limits tends to be the pace at which you can continue moving during a run of marathon proportions.

This is not to say that the easy aerobic feel of the MAP or the compelling, more formidable experience of the SAP are not important. All the zones have meaning and significance. In fact, when I am participating in a multiday event, I run most of the race in my MAP. I might, for strategic reasons, jump into a bit of SAP when I feel the timing is right, such as when I want to break the spirit of a close competitor and gain the upper hand in a psychological battle. The reason I emphasize the importance of the MEP is because it is such a powerful monitoring tool and a key to making steady and everlasting progress. By consistently moving in this narrow ten-beat band, you will be able to keep track of the changes you make—both good and bad—and generate greater productivity at an effort level that can be maintained. While the MEP can be powerful, it can also be elusive. It may require a bit more refining and cultivating than the other two cardio c-quences. While the MAP and SAP zones become readily apparent once you are attuned to their visual, auditory, and kinesthetic characteristics, the MEP might need to be tweaked a bit, but it is well worth it. Fine-tuning and adjusting this cardio c-quence (target training zone) is your most important initial focus. In fact, when you first begin your cardio c-quence training program, your primary objective is to make sure that your MEP zone is set correctly. I will show you how to do that in the next chapter. Once I adjust the MEP zone, up or down, it will necessitate similar up or down adjustments in the MAP and SAP zones as well.

Sensory anchors:

In the MEP, there is a vigilant monitoring of each sensory channel as the sights, sounds, and feelings relate to the task at hand. Your mind is asking your body what information it needs to know to most efficiently and effectively get the job done.

Visual anchors:

The visual images of the MEP are predominantly external. The world looks clear and defined. There is a sense of being in "real-time" when you are in the MEP—unlike the SAP, where images seem to speed up and whiz by, or the MAP, where visual information seems to lazily float by.

Auditory anchors:

Auditory information in the MEP, like its visual counterparts, is precise and definite. While most of the auditory stimuli you listen for will pertain to the task at hand, you will be able to access other sounds as well. In the productive MEP, you hear the sounds you make as you go about your task. You monitor the sound of your breathing, keeping it under control and manageable. You listen for telltale signals that indicate how well you are performing. These can be the quality of the sound as your feet make contact with the ground, as you shift the gears on your bike, or as your arm glides into the water and the start of each swim stroke. You learn to make the necessary adjustments based on the sounds you hear—placing your foot more gently on the ground, a more delicate hand on the gear changer, greater relaxation in your arms as they come out of the water.

Kinesthetic anchors:

You feel totally connected to your body, blending just the right blend of body awareness, attention to the environment, and focus on the movement. You feel productive and prolific, able to get the job done without losing touch with the process.

RPE index:

On a scale of zero to ten, where zero is the absolute easiest you ever exercised and ten is the absolute hardest you ever went (you can't go anymore), your MEP sessions should be between five and seven.

Breathing:

You may notice that your breathing starts to rise up in your chest and the sound of a slight forced expulsion of air appears. However, you are able to control your breathing and both bring it down and quiet it down relatively easily.

Mindset:

While performing your MEP sessions, you want to feel as if you are moving with the awareness of tightrope walker: balanced, in control, and totally aware of what is happening in your body. If you relax too much, the internal images in your mind can absorb you, causing you to daydream and lose touch with the present and the world all around you. This loss of connection can induce you to lose your sense of balance on this high wire strung between the comfortable MAP and the challenging SAP. Similarly, becoming too fanatical about pushing the pace and driving yourself to the limit and beyond can also create instability. You want your focus to be on the way your body feels, not on trying to push yourself as hard as you can. You are not striving to go all out, you are consciously holding something back, of going to the edge of but not beyond it.

YOUR SPEEDY ANAEROBIC PACE (SAP)

The SAP represents the other end of the energy-producing spectrum in which you are burning sugar. The speedy anaerobic pace is up-tempo, challenging, and one notch above the MEP but not quite an all-out or flight-or-fight frenzy, where you just put your head down and explode forward. The SAP is more controlled than that and can represent the final stage of a balanced physical-training program. Once you build an aerobic fat-burning foundation, learn how to get in touch with your body, and develop an efficient and productive movement style, you might choose to include SAP interval training as regular feature of your weekly training routine. SAP sessions stimulate the body's anaerobic sugar-burning muscle fibers and help prepare you to withstand the rigors of unexpected and demanding physical challenges. I often recommend SAP workouts when I prepare a client for an event such as a 10K, half-marathon, marathon, or ultra. I only do so, however, if my client has consistent energy levels, is injury-free, and continues to be excited by and look forward to this the more rigorous and challenging style of training.

Visual anchors:

As you move into the SAP, the dimensionality and depth of the visual world changes. The world begins to flatten out and become more two-dimensional. The peripheral expansiveness gives way to a "tunneling" of your vision. The world begins to look as if you are running through a tunnel with the scenery painted on the inside walls. You may become aware that you are starting to stare at a spot in front of you, often down and to the right or left. Internal visual images are no longer easily accessible to you. You have to concentrate on what you are doing in order to keep moving. There is no way you have even one moment to spare to let your mind wander as it did in the MAP. This is the visual world of the SAP.

Auditory anchors:

You notice the sound of the forced expulsion of air, which now permeates all auditory stimuli. You can't get away from it. You may learn to control it better, but it is always there, in the background somewhere. No longer are sounds distinct and various. They start to blur together and lose their distinctiveness. What was once a soothing blend of natural melodies woven together in a harmonic quilt has now become a cacophony. The auditory information is now close-in, enveloping, and, to some, nearly suffocating. The sound of your breathing, of your feet hitting the ground, become the primary auditory inputs, along with that little voice inside your head that is screaming, "Keep going. Don't stop."

Kinesthetic anchors:

There is a feeling of urgency, even alarm, in the SAP. You may begin to feel the need to shift your weight forward, perhaps landing more on the front of your foot than the back. When this happens, relax as best you can. Breathe as deeply as possible. Emphasize the heel-to-ball motion of the foot. Feel the butterflies fluttering in your hands; the rose pedals in the corner of your mouth. Stay focused; keep moving forward. You can expect a change in your perception of the world as you enter the SAP cardio c-quence. Instead of a feeling at one with the world around you, you will probably begin to feel distinct and separate, as though you are running through and past the objects that surround you. You are no longer part of the environment. You are yourself, alone, striving to survive. Your attempts to rush through time—to make time disappear—only make it seem as if time is starting to stand still. You want it to end. Your commitment is to be strong and powerful—a force to be reckoned with. There is no time to let your mind wander, only time to get the job done. The SAP exists because you must survive and protect yourself. You will not let anyone take advantage of you. You are intent on leaving your mark on the world. The SAP is your statement of power, but, as the wisdom of the ages suggests, for power to be effective, it must be wielded judiciously.

RPE index:

On a scale of zero to ten, where zero is the absolute easiest you ever exercised and ten is the absolute hardest you ever went (you can't go any more), your SAP sessions will ideally range from between seven and nine.

Breathing:

During your SAP sessions, you will notice that your breathing moves higher in the chest and becomes considerably more rapid; you hear a forced expulsion of air.

Mindset:

Your SAP sessions should be up-tempo, exciting, and rigorous but not out of control and panicked. You will find it very difficult to carry on a conversation or let your mind wander. You must stay focused on what you are doing. Time seems to slow down to a crawl, passing by at an agonizingly slow pace. While you are getting plenty accomplished, the effort you are engaged in certainly is not sustainable for an extended period.

Energy levels:

Because of its reliance on sugar-based energy production, the SAP can promote a destabilization of your energy levels. This does not have to be the case. As long as you follow the recommended proportion of MAP, MEP, and SAP cardio c-quences in your training schedule, eat balanced and wholesome meals, and be receptive to the experience your body is having, you can reap the benefits of the up-tempo SAP workout and suppress the negative downside. You might notice that after SAP sessions your energy levels may be somewhat lower than when you started or while you were working out. That is okay and can be expected. Unlike the MAP, which ideally relies on the body's copious fat stores as the main source of energy, the SAP draws from the limited sugar banks. The energy lows that can accompany the SAP workouts can be managed by having a well-balanced meal after the session. I recommend waiting about thirty to forty-five minutes, no longer than an hour, before you begin a well-balanced meal. Until then, concentrate on getting rehydrated by sipping water. Consider performing SAP workouts at the end of the day to protect yourself against the possibility that your energy level may go down after you are done. If your SAP training is positioned at the end of the day as opposed to the start of it, you will be in a better position to do something about it—like rest and get some nourishment!

As time goes on, I want you to notice that you are able to get more accomplished in each of the zones without feeling as if you have to work harder to do it. Imagine this, for example: when you first start the training program, you go on a treadmill and gradually increase its speed and elevation until you are in the recommended MEP target heart-rate zone. You notice that in order to keep your heart rate in the MEP, the treadmill might have to be set at a four-mile-per-hour pace. After four to six weeks of following the schedule and keeping your heart rate within the your recommended cardio c-quences, you begin to notice that at the same heart rate—indeed the same level of effort—you are now jogging at four-and-a-half miles per hour. Six weeks later you are at five miles per hour, and it still feels the same as when you started and you were walking a full mile an hour slower. This is the promise that lies ahead for you with the cardio c-quence training system: getting more accomplished without having to force yourself to work harder.

17

Meet Your New Training Buddy:
A Heart-Rate Monitor

A heart-rate monitor will become your training buddy when you begin the cardio c-quence program. If you already own a monitor, I will show you how to use it for maximum benefit. If you're just about to buy one, be prepared to spend from about $89 to $199. Heart-rate monitors usually consist of two pieces: a belt and a watch. The elastic transmitter belt straps around your chest and picks up the electrical impulses created by the pumping of the heart. The belt then sends a wireless radio signal to a receiver, usually a watch that displays this information as a digital heartbeats per minute (bpm) reading on its face. Amazing! When I first ran with a heart-rate monitor in the mid-1980s, the cumbersome early models consisted of a box that I fastened to my chest with an ace bandage. The sleek new models have become my favorite running companion.

When shopping for a heart-rate monitor, choose from a well-known company. Make sure that the equipment is backed up by a knowledgeable and supportive technical staff. The most well-known manufacturer is Polar Electro. Other companies include Acumen, CardioWatch, and Freestyle. There are even monitors that talk to you through a headset. You will probably do well with any of them. As with most electronic products, you get what you pay for, and nowhere is this more fitting than with a heart-rate monitor. Buy from a reputable company, and beware of cheap bargain brands.

In most instances, there is no need to purchase a top-of-the-line model. The technology remains fairly constant from model to model, the main difference being the additional bells and whistles such as memory, timers, alarms, night-light, and multiple-zone settings. I highly recommend you get a programmable monitor. You will want to set upper and lower limits to the receiver so that it signals you when you are out of the preset target zone. Other desirable features are time of day, stop watch, and a night-light for those predawn or late evening runs. An additional feature I employ quite a lot is a timer—a function that you'll need to when you begin to incorporate speedy anaerobic pace interval training into your program. The timer can be set to trigger an alarm at whatever interval sequence you desire. In other words, you can set the timer to activate an alarm for whatever length of time you want the rest and recovery cycles to be. Most sporting-goods stores and running-specialty shops carry monitors. Check the Internet for the widest variety of model selection and pricing options.

Whenever you use a monitor, make sure all the elements are in place so you get an accurate reading.

Check your belt and transmitter:

As you perspire, your heart-rate monitor belt can stretch and lose contact with the skin, causing wide fluctuations of the heart rate. Make sure the belt is pulled snugly to create the slightest bit of tension against your chest. The electrodes on the transmitter belt must remain in contact with your skin in order to keep sending a signal to the receiver belt. If the belt is too loose, it will lose contact with the skin, and the transmission of information to the receiver watch will be interrupted. This will cause the monitor to give off inaccurate readings. I've seen numbers as low as 0 and as high as 240 appear during a training session. When numbers this extreme appear on your watch, it usually means that your belt wasn't set up correctly. I get quite a lot of calls from concerned clients who see these unexpectedly high or low readings when they are training and want to know if something is wrong with them. Once they tighten the belt, as I suggest, the problem usually disappears.

Wear your belt so the logo is facing up. Putting the belt on upside down—or in the wrong position on your chest (it belongs in the center of your chest, right across your ribcage)—can also affect the accuracy of the monitor.

When the heat or humidity is high or during challenging workouts when you might be sweating a lot, try wearing your transmitter belt over your T-shirt. Your heart rate will be picked up through a damp shirt. Placing the belt on the outside of your shirt under these conditions stabilizes the belt and eliminates heart-rate fluctuations. It also eliminates the possibility of surface abrasions and skin irritations that can affect people with sensitive skin. Remember your shirt must be damp for this strategy to work effectively.

Under dry conditions, with little humidity in the air, moisten the part of the belt directly under the electrode transmitters at the start of your workout. The moisture provides the best contact between the electrodes and your skin. I suggest using water rather than saliva, which for some odd reason has become the custom. Water is more sanitary, especially when belts are shared among friends and family. I always finish my working by wiping the belt off with an alcohol-soaked cotton pad to keep it extra clean.

Keep track of how long you have used the monitor. The lithium batteries in both the transmitter and receiver have to be replaced periodically (about every two to three years). Most manufacturers require that you send back the transmitter and receiver for battery replacement and servicing. Check with your manufacturer or dealer for instructions on what to do.

Beware of the drift:

Heat and dehydration can elevate your heart rate. This is especially true when training in severe heat, humidity, or direct sunlight. You can expect your heart rate to go as high as five, ten, or even twenty beats above your zone without significant changes in the way you feel. As you become acclimated to the heat, your heart rate will likely return to more typical levels as long as you take precautions to stay hydrated, wear a light-colored (preferably white) hat and shirt, sunglasses, and use sunscreen to keep direct sunlight off your body.

Remain fully hydrated:

Since dehydration can elevate your heart rate and cause the readings to be much higher than expected, adequate hydration is essential. Constantly sip water throughout the day, especially when the heat or humidity could be a concern. Do not guzzle a big bottle all at once before you are ready to roll. Be mindful of the need to constantly and gently saturate the cells of your body with water. This means having a bottle of water by your side and taking small sips throughout the day as opposed to big doses at well-spaced intervals. As a general rule, drink at least one-half your body weight in ounces of water every day. Sip on water before, during, and after your movement sessions. You'll know if you're sufficiently hydrated if your urine is plentiful and clear.

Before we move on, I want to be clear that the monitor is just a piece of equipment that provides information about your heart. Simply wearing a monitor isn't going to make a difference in your training. Just knowing your heart rate is not empowering. You don't just want to harness yourself to the monitor and repeatedly discover how high you can get your heart rate (one of the many strategies I have seen used by neophyte heart-rate monitor aficionados). Nor do you want to just look at the numbers that pop up on the screen. What is empowering is being present to the entire complex of sights, sounds, and feelings associated with a given heart-rate range. Be open to your total experience, not just the numbers on your monitor, and you will be unstoppable as you move from where you are toward the possibility of who you can be.

18

Create a Customized Training Program

Like the music teacher who asks his student to rehearse his scales, I am asking you to commit yourself to a training schedule for at least eight to twelve weeks. Both the aspiring musician and you share the goal of being so at one with the instrument, in this case your body, that you achieve just the right rhythm and tempo to create a masterful and magnificent performance. The way to get there is through practice and repetition.

The training program that follows can vary in complexity, from a simple "go out and move in a state you enjoy" to the more complex weekly pattern of different cardio c-quences. You can follow the program I outline, or you can, through time, create your own based upon your expanding sense of what works for your body.

Before I get into how to decide which cardio c-quences to use and how often to use them, I want to emphasize one point: part of me wants to tell you it absolutely doesn't matter what you do as long as you move regularly and comfortably in an aerobic fat-burning state. As my life becomes more demanding in terms of time and pressure, I gravitate to a daily routine of MAP aerobic runs because I enjoy the sense of calm and peacefulness they bring. At certain times, that is all I want and all I seek. At other times, when my business demands are manageable and my personal life is under control, I'm up to the challenge of mixing in some MEPs and a SAP. I have learned not to force myself into the more stressful SAP training routines when my life is providing more than enough anaerobic-like challenges. Business travel is a great example. While one of my greatest passions is working one-on-one with clients at seminars, I do not enjoy the travel component of extended business trips. I once did, but that was before I was married, had a family, and air travel seemed more exciting. Now, I'm often gone for weeks on end, living out of a suitcase, and dashing from plane connection to taxi to my next appointment. Under these conditions, I already experience plenty of anaerobic sugar-burning stress in my day-to-day life. Why add more? When I do get to carve out an hour here and there for a movement session, I do only what my body wants and enjoys. Sometimes, that means jogging at a twelve-minute-per-mile pace along a highway or preferably a lakeside path where I can wave to all the people as they run by me.

I am always seeking to balance the stressful and challenging sugar-burning moments of my life with calm and relaxing fat-burning movement. Conversely, when I find myself settling into a regular, manageable routine, I thoroughly enjoy spicing up my training with more intense sessions. Even when it comes to performance, training harder—or more—does not necessarily lead to better. Often "better" emerges from where you least expect it. In this case, caring and nurturing your body can produce results in ways that punishing your body can't. As long as whatever you do brings you more in touch with your body—as long as you use each and every movement experience to create a better relationship between you and your body—you are headed in the right direction. Don't let the details of any training system distract you from the big picture, which is to get you to move, feel great about your body, and create exciting new possibilities for your life.

The program options I'm about to outline are based on years of personal and professional experience and have worked for thousands of people. But if you, like me, sometimes find yourself in a situation where all you want to do is move easily and enjoy the feeling of getting out and taking a break from a busy hectic life, just do it. Not every workout has to lead to something. There's no need to think of everything I outline as an absolute structure to which you must adhere to in order to succeed. The training program is my way of guiding you beyond limiting beliefs of what you may be capable of doing—and for how long you can do it. In the end you and only you can be your own master. I can only impart the wisdom that my own explorations have provided me and offer you support as you proceed along the journey that is your own.

Adjust Your Target Heart-Rate Zones

During the start of your cardio c-quence training program, your primary objective is to make sure that your zones are set correctly. Remember, neither mathematical formulas nor the gas analyzer and blood lactate tests are foolproof in determining your best target zones. This is especially true of the MEP, because there is so much person-to-person variation. The absolute best method I know of setting a client's MEP zone is for me to run alongside of him or her. After nearly three hundred thousand miles of running, I can tell immediately which zone a person is in as he or she moves. As you might guess, this methodology places quite a premium on my time and limits the amount of people with whom I can work. So I have created a simple exercise for adjusting the cardio c-quences you have already set. You'll need to go through a process of checking your sensory-based experiences in the zones and adjust them up or down accordingly.

To perform this exercise, you'll need about thirty to forty minutes of your time and your heart-rate monitor. Take about two to four minutes for each step. Here's how it goes.

Step 1.

Start off by walking easily with your arms by your side, shoulders relaxed, looking straight ahead. Concentrate on breathing comfortably. You want your breathing to start out low in your belly. Imagine a triangle formed by your hips and your belly button. Inside of the triangle is a "ball." As you breathe in, fill the "ball" up with air so that it gets bigger as you inhale, smaller as you exhale. Feel the "ball" expand as the air comes in, and deflate as the air goes out.

Step 2.

Move your awareness to the ground. Feel the energy flow from the back of your foot to the front of your foot. Have your heel be the first part of your foot that makes contact with the ground. Feel your entire body weight being supported by your heel. Shift your body weight forward. Feel your body weight shifting forward over the arch to the front of your foot. Feel your heel lift up off of the ground as your body weight moves all the way to the front of your foot; your toes begin to spread out, and your entire foot finally leaves the ground. Be aware of the feeling you have as your foot rolls from the back to the front, from your heel to the ball of your foot. The motion is from heel to ball and back to front as you move forward, breathing to the "ball" encased in the triangle formed by your hips and your belly button.

Imagine you are standing on top of the world and this big round sphere is lazily rotating toward you. Lift your feet up just enough to let the earth pass beneath you. Begin to sense that you are not moving toward objects but that the things you see are moving toward you. The world around you seems to be floating by, at its own gentle rate.

Step 3.

Move your arms up so that they are in "dinosaur arm position," with your wrists above your elbows. Your hands are slightly closed and relaxed. Remember the butterflies. Feel the butterflies fluttering on the inside of your hands. Keep your arms close to your body as they swing easily forward and back. Feel the gentle pressure of your arms as they ever so lightly brush against the side of your body. Keep moving as you breathe to the "ball." Feel the energy flow from the back of your foot to the front of your foot, with your arms bent at the elbows holding butterflies in your hands.

Step 4.

Gradually increase your effort as you move. Take your time; don't rush. Over the course of the next two to four minutes, gradually increase your pace. Check your breathing. Maintain contact with the visual world around you. Listen for as many sounds as possible. Note the depth and dimensionality of the visual world. See the peripheral expansiveness in your field of vision. Be aware that you can look straight ahead yet still see objects out to the sides. Observe the differences in the textures of the objects all around you; hear the sound of your feet making contact with the ground. Get in touch with how you are feeling. Note the degree of tension and relaxation throughout your body. Are you comfortable and relaxed, or do you feel pressured and tense? If you can identify areas of tension and pressure, release them, breathe to them, and let yourself go—feel the flow.

Maintain contact with your body and the world around you. Stay at this point. Enjoy these sensations for the moment. Check your watch. What does it say? You should be in your MAP zone.

Are the readings congruent with what you predicted? Are they higher than you expected? Lower? Or are they about the same? Make a mental note.

Step 5.

Bring your intensity level up a notch, and begin to move out of your comfortable aerobic, fat-burning MAP into the more challenging anaerobic sugar-burning SAP cardio c-quence. As you gradually increase your effort, be conscious of the changes in your breathing. Note how your breathing becomes more shallow and rapid as you start to work harder. Listen for the forced expulsion of air. These are all indicators that you have moved into the sugar-burning realm of anaerobic energy production. This forced expulsion of air is your body's way of getting rid of the large carbon dioxide that is produced as your body breaks down sugar to produce energy; it is one of the most notable auditory clues that your energy-producing state is changing.

Look for other visual, kinesthetic, and auditory signals. External visual images will begin to collapse inward and flatten out, reducing your field of vision. The world seems to lose its peripheral expansiveness and three-dimensionality. Objects begin to speed up and whiz past, no longer meandering along at an even, steady flow. You seem to move past objects; objects are no longer floating by you. You no longer can easily access internal images. Daydreaming is not part of the anaerobic world of survival. What do you listen for? Your body seems to be making more noise than the rest of the world. You hear the sound of your feet hitting the ground, the air blowing past your ears, your arms brushing against the side of your body. What can you feel? The heightening sense of urgency and alarm as you begin to strain to keep increasing the pace. Your chest begins to tighten, shoulders become tense, and your body shifts forward so that the initial contact with the ground now becomes the front of your foot, not the back; the ball rather than the heel.

Once these sights, sounds, and feelings manifest themselves, you are in the SAP. Check your watch. Where is your heart rate? Is it in the SAP? Good. Then you can be pretty confident that you know when you are in the sugar-burning zone.

Step 6.

What if you experience these changes and your heart-rate range is in the MEP? Then the MEP is probably set too high and needs to be lowered. If this is the case, drop your MEP by five beats. Ease up a bit. Bring your heart rate just below the point at which the sugar-burning sensory markers appear. You want the visual world to expand outward once again and the breathing to slow down, become quiet, and fall lower in your belly. You want a sense of efficiency and control to replace the feeling of urgency and alarm that exists in the sugar-burning world. If lowering your heart rate by five beats doesn't do it, after another two to four minutes, bring your heart rate down again by five beats and keep doing so until you are certain you are safely harbored within the MEP zone. You are striving to find shelter in a place just below the point that triggers the SAP-related changes. Once you discover this safe haven, nestle in and hold your position. Give each change in effort at least two to four minutes to stabilize.

What do you do if you arrive at a heart rate that you thought would elicit an anaerobic SAP experience and to the best of your sensory judgment you seem aerobic? The world around you is still three-dimensional and expansive; your breathing continues to be quiet and low to the belly; and you hear sounds up close and far away. You feel no sense of urgency and alarm, and you can dream about whatever pops into your head. If that is the case, raise your heart-rate zones. Again, do this in five-beat increments, every two to four minutes, until you finally elicit the desired state change. Once you begin to see, hear, and feel the telltale signs of anaerobic sugar-burning, you know you are entering the domain of the SAP cardio c-quence. Drop below the point at which you begin to be aware of the forced expulsion of air, the flattening out of the visual world, the loss of range and distinctiveness in your hearing, and the increased feeling of urgency and alarm, and you are once again in your MEP. Adjust your zones up or down accordingly.

Use this method of collaboration between your personal experience and heart-rate response to transform your target heart-rate training schedule from a good guess to a great fit. If your experience of the zone is incongruent with the cardio c-quence descriptions, you must adjust the cardio c-quence zone accordingly. Raise or lower the zone in five-beat increments only and, again, only after you've stabilized your heart rate for at least two to three minutes.

Your Individual Workouts: Putting Theory into Practice

With your zones correctly set, it's time to outline the components of your individualized workout program. You're already familar with the three cardio c-quences in terms of what they look, sound, and feel like. Let us now incorporate them into actual training sessions. Each cardio c-quence workout has a definitive structure and needs to be implemented in its own special way.

Your Warmup and Cool-Down

Spend the first seven to fifteen minutes of your training session asking your body to produce energy slowly. The more gradually you bring your heart rate up, the richer in fat your fuel source will be. As mentioned earlier, by asking your body to produce energy at a nonemergency rate, you increase the likelihood that it will get its energy from fat. When you demand your body produce energy suddenly, it will get its energy from sugar.

Your body stores sugar—the fuel of choice for igniting emergency responses—in the blood, or as glycogen in the muscle and liver. Your anaerobic, fast-twitch sugar-burning muscle fibers have immediate access to these sugar stores and use them to fuel flight-or-fight activity. On the other hand, your body has a much different system for storing the fat, its peacetime fuel. It locks fat away in storage vaults far from the muscles. Since your aerobic, slow-twitch fat-burning muscle fibers produce energy in a controlled and deliberate manner, there is no need to keep the fat reserves in a state of alert. Fat that is not immediately needed for energy is put away for long-term storage. To get at this fat, your body must go through a "fat-mobilization" process before its fat stores can be converted into energy by the aerobic, slow-twitch fat-burning muscle fibers. Mobilizing fat involves a sequence of events that transforms stored body fat into free fatty acids, which are carried by the blood to the aerobic, slow-twitch fat-burning muscle fibers. It takes between seven and fifteen minutes for your body to mobilize fat. Giving your body time to transform its out-of-the-way fat stores into a utilizable fuel can be one of the most effective strategies for ensuring greater reliance on fat as an energy source during your workout and throughout your day.

Ease into your workout. By starting out slowly and bringing your heart rate up gradually, you encourage your body to burn fat right from the start of your movement session. When you burn fat, you keep your sugar stores intact and ensure optimal functioning of your nervous system, better decision making, and a steady stream of energy throughout the day.

The cool-down is simply your warmup in reverse. During the cool-down phase of your training session, you want your heart rate to drop down to nearly as low as it was when you were in your fat-mobilization zone. This is important. Most people I know skip this portion of the workout even more often than the warm-up. The cool-down helps your body transition from an active state into a more sedentary one. The cool-down lets your body redirect the flow of blood away from the large working muscles and back to the internal organs and brain. I am particularly fond of the imagery of the body shifting around blood to provide a greater volume to the essential working muscles. Your body shunts blood by expanding the blood vessels in the large working muscles involved in the motion and constricting the blood vessels in muscle groups and organs that are not immediately needed.

This is how your body delivers more oxygen and nutrient-rich blood to the muscles that need it. However, only your arteries—the blood vessels that carry the blood from your heart to the muscles—have the capacity to dilate and constrict. The veins—the blood vessels that return "spent" blood from the muscles back to the heart and lungs for detoxification and reoxygenation—cannot act like arteries. They do not have muscles that enable them to dilate or constrict. They can expand when the volume of blood sent through them increases due to arterial dilation, but once thus engorged with blood, they need time to shrink and get the "spent" blood out and back to the lungs. You do not want this blood "pooling" in your veins. Spent blood is oxygen-depleted and full of toxic by-products such as lactic acid and carbon dioxide. The faster you get rid of these by-products, the better you will feel. The best way to facilitate the removal of potentially irritating blood is to mechanically pump it out by gently moving the muscles in the same motion you just did.

Your warmup and cool-down can last anywhere from seven to fifteen minutes, depending on the intensity of your cardio c-quence on that day. For instance, when your workout calls for a comfortable, aerobic MAP, your warmup might be between seven to ten minutes, as opposed to a longer twelve to fifteen minutes for the more intense SAP session. When doing a MEP, your warmup and cool-down can be between ten and twelve minutes. It is challenging to allocate time to the warmup and cool-down. For so many of my clients, trying to shoehorn in another fifteen minutes here and ten minutes there into an already hectic life is not easy. It is worth it, though. You'll feel better as you get into your training session, and you will dramatically reduce the prospects of getting stiff and tight. You will feel looser and more flexible, less tense and sore. You will truly look forward to training sessions because you will be certain that they can make you feel great—the outcome we all want.

Stick with the recommended warmup and cool-down for at least four to six weeks or for as long as it takes to get a sense of what is right for you. Almost everyone I work with acquires a "feel" for his own body and can sense when to begin kicking the effort up a notch. Until that time comes, however, stay with the program as designed. Remember, the ultimate objective is for you to compose your own physical masterpiece.

YOUR MOSTLY AEROBIC PACE (MAP)

MAP sessions always begin with a seven-to-ten-minute warm-up, during which time you bring your heart rate up slowly. Take your time. Keep your heart rate in the scheduled target zone. Anywhere in the zone is okay as long as the movement feels comfortable and relaxed. If your heart rate rises above your scheduled zone, slow down. If your heart rate drops below your scheduled zone and that's where your body wants to be, just stay there. In your MAP you're not really required to reach a minimum threshold. Your focus is on the flow of the movement, feeling comfortable, and enjoying the process of moving. If you want to increase or decrease the intensity level in order to stay within the target zone, make adjustments as smoothly as possible. Avoid suddenly speeding up or slowing down. All changes must occur within the smallest increments possible. When trying to keep in the zone by regulating your pace (speed) or mode (walking, jogging, or running), remember the metaphor of sailing a ship versus driving a car. Unlike the car driver, who can accelerate quickly and jam on the brakes, the ship's captain must not suddenly increase or decrease speed. The MAP is your most health-promoting and healing cardio c-quence. Go there for as long and as often as you like. You can walk or run—do whichever you feel like, as long as you stay comfortable, flowing, and in the prescribed zone. Once you are able to run in the MAP, you will begin to experience the phenomenon of running faster and faster, all the while remaining comfortable, aerobic, and fat-burning.

MAP runs can be performed two to four times a week for twenty to sixty minutes at a time, depending on your starting level or time commitment. This does not include the seven-to-ten-minute warmup and cool-down. The duration of the MAP can be extended as long as the heart rate stays in the MAP zone. Increase time in the zone gradually, around twenty minutes every other week, if you wish.

YOUR MOST EFFICIENT PACE (MEP)

MEP sessions always begin with a ten-to-twelve minute warmup. Be efficient, alert, and focused in the MEP. The experience of the MEP is one of heightened awareness. The key is to be steady and in control. Unlike the MAP, where anywhere in the zone is okay, aim to be right in the middle of the zone if possible.

Depending on your goals and aerobic training, you may increase the duration of your MEP every other week for one weekend run only. With some clients, I include a MEP run of a specific distance rather than of a particular duration. This strategy helps to prepare you for a recreational or competitive event. By using a distance as opposed to a duration, you can better gauge changes in pace as your training program progresses. One method involves tracking mile splits over the course of these longer MEP distance runs. A mile split simply means the amount of time it takes you to cover a given mile-long segment of your run.

Ideally, you want your mile splits to be fairly even—your pace for your first mile should be similar to your middle and last mile.

The point of these fortnightly workouts is not to see how fast you can run but how efficient you can be while your heart rate stays within the MEP zone. The same speeding-up phenomenon we mentioned in the MAP discussion applies here as well. Gradually you will notice that you will be moving faster and faster in the MEP zone, while your heart rate and general effort level remain the same. Once again, you will be training your body to move faster and to be more productive without working any harder. This is the best sign of progress you can have.

YOUR SPEEDY ANAEROBIC PACE (SAP)

SAP sessions are modeled after conventional interval training strategy except that we use time (duration) instead of a distance. Interval training sessions are simply an up-tempo bout of exercise for a specified period, followed by an easy recovery segment, usually of the same duration. During your SAP sessions, you will be given a prescribed amount of time within which to stay above the middle zone MEP—a training interval—followed by a recovery period below the MEP of the same duration in your MAP. In effect you will be continually passing through the middle zone to go from SAP to MAP and back again.

Organizing your SAP workouts this way can actually be fun. Set your heart-rate monitor for the upper and lower limits of the MEP cardio c-quence. Once this is done, whenever you enter the SAP zone, the heart-rate monitor alarm will go off, producing a signal that says you are out of the MEP zone and indicating that you have entered the SAP cardio c-quence. When the SAP interval is completed, ease up and allow yourself to slow down and recover. You want your heart rate to pass through the MEP cardio c-quence on its way down to the MAP. As your heart rate does this, the alarm will go from an audible signal (usually a beep), indicating you are above the MEP in the SAP zone, to silence, indicating you are now passing through the MEP zone. Finally, if you let yourself slow down and recover properly, the alarm will be triggered once again as you enter the MAP zone below the lower limit of the MEP. In effect, what you are doing during your SAP session is passing through the middle zone MEP and running from MAP to SAP or "beep to beep." I often call the SAP workout "running through the zone" or "chasing the beep."

The duration of the up-tempo challenges and recoveries change from SAP workout to SAP workout; so do the actual number of repeats. SAP intervals can range from one to five minutes, followed by a recovery period of the same length or less. During a twelve-week program, the sequence goes from one-minute intervals during week one to three-minute intervals during week two to one-and-a-half-minute intervals during week three to five-minute intervals during week four. On week five the same 1–3–1.5–5 minute sequence in repeated over the next four weeks, this time increasing the number of intervals by at least one. (Refer to the chart on the next page: 12-week speedy anaerobic pace training schedule.) At the end of the second four-week period, the entire process is repeated, again in the 1–3–1.5–5 minute sequence with at least one additional interval added each successive week.

By the end of this twelve-week training cycle, I suggest you either go back to week one or increase the number of repeats in the same pattern as in the earlier four-week cycles. I strongly recommend that you do not go beyond twelve weeks without taking a prolonged break from SAP interval training. I find that quarterly schedule changes work best in keeping progress steady and motivation high. This might mean, for instance, that at the completion of your twelve-week schedule, you drop SAP training for the next three months. You will learn to judge this best for yourself. You do not want to get to the point where you begin to dread the SAPs. This can happen if you do not let your body take a break. When the right mix of MAP, MEP, and SAP cardio c-quences are blended together, most of my clients seem to look forward to them. There is a rhythm to the week that begins to set in and feel right. In order for this to happen, though, breaks need to be built in so that you do not begin to feel trapped in a cycle of training that lasts forever.

SAP training hints:

You must be able to recover from the SAP effort and have your heart rate return to the MAP before resuming the up-tempo challenge of the SAP. If your heart rate does not return to the MAP during the recovery period, you must ease off a bit during the SAP segment. You will probably have to jog slowly—or even walk—during the first few SAP recovery segments before your body gets the hang of it.

12-WEEK SPEEDY ANAEROBIC PACE (SAP) INTERVAL TRAINING SCHEDULE

Week Number	Time of Training Intervals (in minutes and seconds)	Time of Recovery Intervals (in minutes and seconds)	Number of Repeats	Total Time of SAP Sessions*
1	1:00	1:00	7	14
2	3:00	3:00	3	18
3	1:30	1:30	6	18
4	5:00	3:00	2	16
5	1:00	1:00	10	20
6	3:00	3:00	4	24
7	1:30	1:30	8	24
8	5:00	3:00	3	24
9	1:00	1:00	13	26
10	3:00	3:00	5	30
11	1:30	1:30	10	30
12	5:00	3:00	4	32

*In minutes; does not include warmup and cool-down.

To Stretch or Not to Stretch

I was once quoted on the front page of *The Wall Street Journal* on the subject of stretching. The *Journal* was intrigued with the fact that I don't advocate stretching. It's not that I don't like to stretch. I just don't believe in the necessity of doing it before I run.

Stretching a cold muscle is the surest way to get injured. I've coached many people who've hurt themselves during a seemingly innocuous stretching routine. It usually happens the day or two before a performance event. Instead of working out, the person decides to stretch. Without a proper warmup, stretching can actually increase the likelihood of getting injured.

Actually, stretching may be a misnomer. You're not stretching a muscle; you're releasing tension to increase the range of motion around a particular joint. A tight muscle doesn't need to be stretched; it needs to be relaxed. I prefer to jettison the term s-t-r-e-t-c-h-i-n-g altogether, for a s-t-r-e-t-c-h-e-d muscle is an injured muscle.

So what should you do to release muscle tension? As you're aware from the muscle-testing chapter, a tense muscle can have nothing to do with the muscle. It can be related to the health of your organs. Tight quadriceps could be related to your small intestines. Hamstring tension could be the result of an imbalance in your digestive system. Muscle testing can help you to consider the big picture.

For most people, the warmup segment of your workout serves the same purpose as stretching. It helps release tension in the muscles involved in movement. Not only are you helping the muscles, you're mobilizing fat. While I don't believe in the need to stretch before a workout, I do believe that flexibility and relaxation exercises can play a role in your training program. How you go about it is essential. The first step is to assume a position that isolates the muscle you want to work on. Isolating a muscle means adopting a position that places gentle pressure on the muscle, which you begin to feel as the muscle starts to tighten. Noticeable tension in the muscle indicates that you've isolated the muscle. Once you isolate it, ease off and use your breathing to release the tension. Feel the air flowing deep into your belly, into the "ball" inside the triangle formed by your hips and belly button. Connect the "ball" to the muscle by imagining the current of air moving from the "ball" to the isolated muscle. Now, as the "ball" expands, so does the muscle. Feel the air expand as you breathe in, and let the air out of the muscle as you breathe out. As you breathe out and the air escapes, release as much tension as possible. Extend the position as you exhale and release tension. Repeat this process, using the breathing to extend the stretch as you exhale. Always avoid forcing yourself to move past the point at which the muscle is tight.

There are two main rules to follow whenever you release tension in a muscle:

1. Always warm up first. This can be accomplished by easy walking, jogging, or any gentle motion that gradually elevates your heart rate.

2. Increase the range of motion when you exhale; never extend a "stretch" while you are holding your breath or inhaling.

RETHINKING WHAT IT MEANS TO WALK

Your body doesn't care if you are walking or running. It wants to move in a particular state, which can be either fat-burning MAP-aerobic, transitional MEP-efficient, or sugar-burning SAP-anaerobic.

The point is to let the state define what you do; don't force a mode (running or walking) when it brings you out of state. If, on a scheduled MAP day, you are particularly tired and worn down and running brings you out of the comfortable fat-burning aerobic state, then slow down and walk. If, on a different day, when you are well-rested and shifting gears from a walk to a run keeps you in state, go with it. The state accommodates the movement, not the other way around. The mode you are moving in is less important than the state in which you are moving. You can walk, jog, or run. It doesn't matter as long as you stay in the desired state. This strategy will apply for every cardio c-quence you do.

At this point in the program, there is only one important distinction we need to make between running and walking. When you are walking, one foot maintains contact with the ground at all times. When you are running, both feet leave the ground for an instant. Other than that, everything is the same. I first noticed this when I went to La Rochelle, France to participate in the indoor six-day world championship. Around the indoor track was a waist-high fence covered with advertising billboards. The first time I left the track to take a break, I looked back toward the track and noticed I couldn't see the participants from the waist down. What next got my attention was the fact that I couldn't tell if the participants were walking or running. The motion was smooth, even, as if the runners skimmed along the surface of the ground, whether they were walking or running. There was hardly any vertical up and down movement of the shoulders; everything seemed to flow horizontally and forward.

There might be one consideration to make regarding the edge that running has on walking. The extra load on the skeletal system created by the impact of the body returning to the ground during the running motion has one distinct advantage. It challenges the bones just enough to keep them strong and better able to maintain bone mineral density. This is especially important in light of the increasing concerns about osteoporosis and the loss of bone mineral density that so many women and men face as they age. My suggestion is to walk or run as long as you stay in the recommended state. The particular mode that is best for you—running or walking—is determined by what your body can do as you keep within the zone. When the time is right, you will run, and once you do, you will open up the possibility that your life will never be the same.

Practice Aerobic Weight Training

I'm a strong advocate of strength training. It's an essential part of a well-rounded fitness program. I've been a regular denizen of weight rooms since high school. As a coach, I see the value of incorporating weights at certain points during a running program. I make sure that my clients start by learning how to move comfortably in their aerobic cardio c-quences before I introduce weight training. However, in most instances I support keeping the muscles toned and strong, with some form of resistance training. The main distinction I make with strength training is similar to the one I make in cardiovascular training. There is strength training that emphasizes anaerobic power and speed outcomes and weight training that produces aerobic endurance outcomes. Anaerobic weight training builds larger, thicker, and more explosive muscles through heavier weights and fewer repetitions. Aerobic weight training creates leaner, more toned muscles with great stamina by relying on a higher number of repetitions and the use of lighter weights. Each style of training accentuates a different muscle fiber. The higher-weight/lower-rep strategy stimulates the anaerobic sugar-burning muscle fibers, causing them to get thicker and denser—a process called hypertrophy of the muscle. The lower-weight/higher-rep strategy of muscular endurance training stimulates the aerobic fat-burning muscle fibers, causing them to increase their capacity to exert a moderate force for a longer and longer duration. A sample aerobic workout would be as follows:

First set:

Warm up with a weight light enough to allow twenty-five to thirty-five repetitions. Concentrate on your form and breathing. Always exhale as you exert the most force (move the weight).

Second set:

Increase the weight and perform twenty to twenty-five reps.

Third set:

Increase the weight again, and perform fifteen to twenty reps, and so on.

Basic strategy:

Increase the weight and drop the repetitions for each successive set.

In terms of body parts, I recommend changing routines every three months. Two to three total body workouts per week is great. You can also split up your strength training sessions into four or five smaller sessions that exercise one to three different body parts each workout. Personally, I never spend more than twenty minutes using weights on any given day. I supplement strength training with five to fifteen minutes of abdominal exercises at least five days per week.

Putting It All Together

With your heart-rate zones in place and an understanding of how the individual and supplemental workouts are structured, you're ready to move into one of three levels of my training program. In level one, comfort is your guide. The goal is to go out and move and enjoy the feeling of your body in motion. Level two still emphasizes aerobic, fat-burning exercise while introducing more focused workouts in which you try to manage your heart rate with a narrow, efficient zone. Level three is for those who enjoy recreational or competitive sports.

Here, I describe each level using the training story of a client. At the end, I list several sample workouts that you can use as a guide to form a training routine that fits your lifestyle in terms of time commitment and personal preferences. For information about more specific 5K, 10K, and marathon training charts, visit my Website at www.worldultrafit.com.

All the clients I have chosen to profile have run a marathon. Feel free to pick and choose the elements of their programs that best relate to your goals. Whichever program you choose, make a promise to yourself that you will have some fun, enjoy the process of moving, and not get too hung up on the outcomes of your efforts. The most powerful outcome is to move as often and as consistently as possible. You'll know you are successful when you feel great in motion, have uniform and abundant energy levels, are excited about what's happening with your body, and look forward to your movement sessions rather than dreading them. I promise that you will be amazed at the energy you create, how much you grow to look forward to your training sessions, and how in the end you get the outcomes you were committed to in the first place. With that pledge in place, we are ready to begin.

Level One: Comfortable, Steady, and Enjoyable

Level-one training is right for a wide range of people—the beginner, just starting to get to know his or her body, the competitive athlete looking for a break in the off-season, or the stressed-out executive who needs to offset a hectic, sugar-burning lifestyle with high-quality, aerobic, fat-burning experiences. Level one can be for the homemaker or college student who enjoys gentle movement each day while listening to music. It can also be for the overweight dad who has been avoiding exercise but is now committed to losing a few pounds, living a healthier lifestyle, and maintaining more reliable energy levels.

Level one moves you into a moderate, aerobic, fat-burning state as often as possible, whenever you can, for as long as it feels right. Level one relies on the MAP cardio c-quence to promote the extensive use of fat as an energy source. Unlike most conventional training procedures, the MAP does not have to hurt to be good for you. The aim is to provide you and your body time to get to know each other and discover how to make each other happy.

Level one has provided an incredible transformation in my own training. I have learned I can kick back and enjoy the experience of running a twelve-minute-per-mile pace instead of a sub-eight-minute pace during my training runs. After more than thirty years of daily running, my body doesn't want to be pushed anymore, and I can live with that. I go out and run in my MAP zone, stay in touch with my body and the experience I am having, and achieve a state of calm. I am moving, my body is happy, and that is all that there needs to be while I am in the MAP. By relying on the MAP experience, level one promotes the adage that the movement itself is the reward.

Ideally, you want to do your MAP workouts as early in the day as possible. Since MAP sessions stimulate greater fat utilization, they enhance the quality of your energy the rest of the day. By getting your body to burn more fat, MAP workouts discourage the use of sugar. This has a stabilizing effect on your blood-sugar level and increases the likelihood that you will have stable, high-quality energy throughout the day.

Commit to a minimum of three to five days per week in the aerobic fat-burning zone. You don't have to stop there, though. Move as often as you like—every day, if possible. You will always benefit from moving in your MAP as long as you are committed to remaining comfortable, aerobic, and fat-burning. For me, running in my MAP is the movement experience I enjoy the most. A few years ago, I was asked by *Runners' World* magazine why I ran twenty miles a day. My answer was simple: I ran twenty miles a day because that's all the time I had.

LEVEL-ONE CLIENT PROFILE

Frank has already achieved what most people dream about: he's built a multimillion dollar business, owns three homes in beautiful areas, and has a loving family. Now, as he approaches his fifties, his priorities have shifted. He has neglected his health on the way to building his business. He doesn't feel strong. He wants to take his body and his health up the level that he's reached in the other aspects of his life. Frank has heard of my work with other Tony Robbins participants and comes to me to set up a program to increase his energy and vitality and achieve a breakthrough in the way he feels.

Frank and I do our first session together in September 1996. He is quizzical; he isn't sure what I can do for a man who hasn't run since he was in the army thirty years earlier. We run and walk for forty-five minutes to one hour, and, as with so many of my clients, Frank is amazed that he feels better at the end of the session than at the beginning. For the next ten months, Frank commits to make regular exercise part of his life. Three days a week, he warms up with a fifteen-minute walk, alternates running and walking in his MAP zone for thirty minutes, and cools down with a fifteen-minute walk. On the weekend, he does one MEP session for about twenty minutes with the same warm-up and cool down. He is fascinated by how simple changes in his arm position, his breathing, and the way his feet relate to the ground can enhance the way he feels as he moves. He is astonished that an increase in his shoe size can make walking and running so much more enjoyable. He particularly loves using the roller-coaster metaphor. He lets himself lose momentum going up the hills, shifting into baby steps, and gains momentum going down the hills as he opens up his stride into a frolicking run.

By August 1997, Frank increases his commitment to walk and run five to six times a week. Frank loves his new ritual of getting up every morning, having a cup of hot water with lemon, and going out for his hour-long run/walk. His investment of time pays tremendous dividends. The rest of day he has more energy, can think more clearly, and is able to remain much calmer in the face of situations that used to stress him out. He begins to realize that what has stopped him from committing an hour a day in the past was his belief that time was too scarce. When he actually allocates the hour, time becomes abundant. His need to rest and recover decreases. He gets up earlier, goes to bed later, and is liberated from his limiting belief that he must get eight hours of sleep every night.

Frank builds up to the point where on January 31, he is able to run/walk for two and half hours, covering a half a marathon. This is the first time he runs continuously for more than thirty minutes. On this particular run/walk, he extends his longest running segment to forty-five minutes. This is the breakthrough that Frank has been looking for and he begins to consider that his dream of running a marathon can actually come true. He asks whether I think he can do the Los Angeles Marathon, which was coming up in six weeks. I tell him, "There's no question in my mind. It's only a matter of whether you want to and whether you're ready to tell others that you're going to run it." Frank decides to step up to the challenge. He announces his intention to his friends, who suggest he is crazy to take on the "pain" they believe running a marathon will bring. I assure him that the dreaded "wall" his friends insist he will run into at twenty miles doesn't have to be there. Once he commits to the race, I recommend he maintain his daily thirty minute MAP run/walk, sandwiched by a fifteen-minute warmup and cool-down. Every other week, he extends his Saturday MEP runs by twenty to thirty minutes. We plan a special dress rehearsal run/walk for four weeks later so he can feel what it's like to be on his feet for three hours or more.

The dress-rehearsal technique, which I use with all my clients who are preparing for an event, is more than just another training run. It allows them to gather, test, and choose which equipment and provisions they'll use on event day. Clothing choices are determined by possible weather conditions. We consider all the possible weather conditions and have the appropriate clothing options ready. Frank gathers the shoes, shorts, tights, a warmup suit, a T-shirt, and hat that we think he might use on marathon day. The objective is to set all this up in advance so on event day, he won't have to think about anything. All he will have to do is grab his bag of provisions and go. By the end of February, he has all his gear set and is ready for a long run that we inspirationally name the "Road to LA" 30K run/walk. It is a particularly cool morning, and Frank wears a polypropylene long-sleeve shirt and shorts underneath loosely fitting warmup bottoms. To prevent chaffing, I suggest calendula ointment under his armpits and groin, and, to Frank's surprise, plastic bandages on his nipples. Even though I know that Frank's fat-burning training and nutritional strategies will minimize his dependency on food for energy during the event, I go along with his insistence that he bring snacks on the run. In a plastic bag in my body pack, I carry bits of celery and carrots, along with almonds that have been soaked in water overnight to soften them up. For fluids, we alternate water and a special "green" drink composed of natural grains and grasses providing easily absorbed minerals and vital nutrients.

We run the February workout together. As is sometimes the case when I run with clients, I decide not to tell Frank in advance what we will do. The strategy starts with our customary fifteen-minute walk, followed by a sixty-minute run, which is the longest nonstop stretch of running he's ever done. We then walk for fifteen minutes and follow up his personal best for a continuous run with a forty-five-minute run, which equals his previous personal best. It's mind-boggling to Frank that he is doing back-to-back runs that are as long as he's previously done before and he still feels great. We shift into a fifteen-minute walk and then graduate into a thirty-minute segment. My plan is to complete the run with fifteen-minute run/walk cycles, but Frank pleads with me to make the next segment thirty minutes, bringing us within a fifteen-minute walk from our final destination. Frank realizes he is about to complete this unbelievable experience, and grabs my cell phone to share his excitement with his wife. He tells her he'll be home in fifteen minutes and asks her to get the Jacuzzi ready and be prepared to go out dancing that night.

Two weeks before the marathon, Frank's daughter and wife come down with the flu, and he takes care of them. By the next week, he comes down with the same symptoms. He wonders out loud whether he should go through with the marathon. I tell him to defer that decision, to focus on getting healthy. If he wakes up on race day and doesn't feel like running, he won't run. If he makes it to the starting line and three miles into the race his body tells him not to continue, he could stop. For the moment he needs to focus on eating well, resting, and drinking lots of fluids. It's been my experience that when illness symptoms occur prior to a big event, as they often do, it can be used as opportunity for us to take the pressure off the performance.

Race morning arrives, and Frank feels well enough to run. Our strategy is to run from aid station to aid station, which are situated one mile apart along the course. I remind Frank that our objective isn't to run twenty-six miles. It's to run one mile twenty-six times. At the eighteen-mile point, which represents the greatest distance that Frank has ever covered to date, we take a planned break. Frank lies down on a bus-stop bench and, as I had done many times previously, I stimulate the gait reflex points on the top, sides, and bottom of his feet to alleviate discomfort and promote greater fluidity of movement. By mile twenty-one, Frank pulls ahead of me with a skipping motion. I catch up to him and ask what's going on. "Why did you take off like that?" I ask. He tells me that he's just realized that the "wall" he's been waiting for the last three miles isn't coming and he can't contain his joy. The last few miles go by swiftly and, for the most part, in silence as Frank savors the completion of his incredible journey which started from scratch a little over a year earlier.

Startup workout:

Fifteen-minute warmup walk, fifteen minutes alternating running and walking in the MAP zone, fifteen-minute cool-down three to four days a week. Total time: forty-five minutes.

Typical weekly routine:

Fifteen-minute warmup walk, thirty minutes in the MAP zone, fifteen-minute cool-down walk three to four days a week with one MEP workout every week. Total time: one hour per workout.

Combination long run/walk:

Fifteen-minute warmup walk, forty-five-minute MEP run, fifteen-minute walk, thirty-minute MEP run, fifteen-minute walk, fifteen-minute MEP run, fifteen-minute cool-down walk. Total time: two and a half hours.

The Road to LA rehearsal run:

Fifteen-minute warmup, sixty-minute MAP run, fifteen-minute walk, forty-five minute MEP run, fifteen-minute walk, thirty-minute MAP run, fifteen-minute walk, thirty-minute MEP run, fifteen-minute cool-down walk. Total time: four hours.

Level Two: Focused, Efficient, and Maintainable

The main objective of level-two training is to increase your efficiency and learn to be more productive as you move. Unlike level one, where the focus is on getting to know your body and transforming it into a better fat burner, level two seeks to train you to get more accomplished without feeling as though you are working any harder.

Level-two training can be a great preparation for a performance event. I have seen recreational and competitive athletes perform at their absolute best while performing two to three MEP training sessions per week supplemented with two to three MAP workouts on alternate days. The key outcome of level two is to increase your productivity in the middle or MEP zone. This means that as time goes by, you will start speeding up in the MEP while you heart rate and sense of effort and intensity remain constant.

This speeding up manifests itself in a variety of ways. You may start out your level-two training by needing to shift from a run to a walk and back again, or having to jog slowly in order to keep your heart rate in the MEP target zone. After a few weeks of level two training, you might notice that you no longer have to break up your MEP sessions by alternating walking and running. You are soon able to stay in the MEP zone by walking less and running more until you reach the point where you can run the entire time.

Once you can run through the entire MEP movement session, you begin to recognize that your pace picks up and you are now running faster and faster in the MEP. Speeding up without having to work harder is the desired MEP outcome. I remember this phenomenon when I was preparing for my thousand-mile race. While running in my MEP target zone of 145 to 155, I reached the point where I could maintain a steady 5:45 pace per mile. I wasn't straining or uncomfortable. To the contrary, I felt surprisingly in control and calm. I remember thinking that my main challenge was to figure out how to get my legs to move quickly enough to keep up with the fabulous amount of energy my body seemed to possess. It was as though I had transplanted a nuclear-powered rocket engine in the chassis of an ordinary automobile. That's how I want you to feel during your MEP runs as you progress through level two.

Level-Two Client Prolile

Jake is one of those men who looks great without doing a lot. You get the feeling that he can do whatever he sets his mind to. Strong and athletic, he tells me he's lost about thirty pounds over the last year because of a big change in his nutritional habits. He's become a vegetarian and reintroduced intense running and weight-training routines modeled on what he'd done as a youth. Still, his energy is not where he wants it to be and he's not as lean as he'd like.

During the run/walk analysis, I lead Jake through the cardio c-quences. I notice that as we move from fat-burning to sugar-burning states, his movement becomes labored and forced. He's strong enough to push himself through, though he looks as if he's straining and tense in the process. Since Jake has already done some running, he quickly picks up the difference between jogging in the easy MAP mode and running in the more focused and productive MEP cardio c-quence.

I conclude that Jake will benefit the most from a schedule that temporarily suspends the high-intensity sugar-burning SAP runs he's been addicted to and alternate comfortable MAP runs with more focused runs in his MEP zone. As I had done with Frank, I schedule bi-monthly combination run/walks that increase by twenty minutes each time.

On days he is scheduled to do a MAP workout, Jake follows his run with twenty minutes of moderate endurance-style weight-training instead of the heavy weight work to which he is accustomed. He works on two to three different body parts during each workout. To build lean, toned muscles suited for endurance activities, I encourage him to perform three to five high-repetition sets for each body part.

Jake completes this first three-month program and is pleased with the changes. His body is leaner, and he has more consistent energy. He wants a new goal. Jake confesses to me that at one time, the thought of doing a marathon had intrigued him but he dismissed it because he associated long-distance running with pain and exhaustion. He couldn't envision running in that state for twenty-six miles. But after completing his initial twelve-week program, the act of running is no longer painful. He has transformed running into something that is much more exhilarating and sustainable. What started out as relatively slow saunter in his target zone has become a noticeably faster run. Emboldened by the realization he is running faster without feeling that he has to work harder, Jake decides to go to the next level and signs up for the Chicago Marathon.

I create a twelve-week program that alternates MAP and MEP workouts throughout each week. On weekends, Jake performs either a combo run/walk or an extended MEP run that starts at sixty minutes and increases by twenty minutes every other week, bringing him to two hours and twenty minutes two weeks before the marathon. His combo run/walks begin at ninety minutes and increase by fifteen to thirty minutes every other week till he peaks at three hours three weeks before the marathon.

Jake gets into his training program with gusto, excited about the possibility of completing his first marathon. He hooks up with a group of runners in his community preparing for the same event. After a few training sessions with them, he calls me to express concern that he might not be training hard enough. The others he knows are running much faster for longer distances and doing intense speed work every week. "Shouldn't I be doing the same?" he asks. I tell him that of course he can if he wants to. It's just that because of his anaerobic sugar-burning background, adding sugar-burning SAP workouts to his routine will more likely break him down than speed him up. The most likely way for him to have a great first marathon experience is to run faster by starting off slower.

So many factors go into running a marathon. If you line up at the start with nagging aches and pains from training too hard and for too long, not only will you create a miserable experience, but you will also dread doing it again—regardless of your time. "What's the statement you want to make as the race ends?" I ask Jake. "Do you want to agonize your way to the finish, only to feel broken and exhausted as soon as it's over? Or, do you want to exquisitely manage your state each and every moment of the event, gaining momentum and excitement you move along?" Jake is certain he wants to finish strong and not have to spend a lot of time recovering from the event. His schedule is too tight, it can't afford the luxury of taking days off or scheduling his meetings around his recreational activities. In fact, Jake has a meeting scheduled for the very next morning after the marathon, not in Chicago, but in Louisville, Kentucky!

I convince Jake that much of the mystique that surrounds the marathon is overblown and exaggerated. It does not have to be the grueling, agonizing, and insufferable event it is often made out to be. While some people seek to glorify pain and misery, Jake wasn't one of them. The day of the event, he stays in his MEP cardio c-quence for most of the race, managing his state and keeping himself out of jeopardy. Jake starts off easy and gains momentum, running a strong second half and coming in jubilant and excited. It turns out he's just a few minutes behind his training buddies, who stagger in as newly sworn members of the "Never again!" gang.

The next morning, Jake hops on the first plane out of Chicago on his way to a 9:00 A.M. breakfast meeting in Kentucky. Jake opens the meeting by thanking everyone for coming and sharing his excitement about running his first marathon the day before. For a second, people think he's kidding because he looks so good. Meanwhile, back in Chicago, his bleary-eyed, broken-down friends are gingerly and hesitatingly walking backward off the curb into their taxis. For a mere gain of 10 minutes, a lifetime of enjoyment is lost. His friends can't imagine running another step. Jake is already talking about his next race.

TYPICAL WEEK DURING A
<u>TWELVE-WEEK TRAINING PROGRAM</u>

Monday, Wednesday, Sunday:

Seven-to-ten-minute warmup, twenty-to-thirty-minute MAP, seven-to-ten-minute cool-down, twenty minutes weights, five minutes abdominal workout. Total time: fifty-nine to seventy-nine minutes.

Tuesday, Thursday, Saturday:

Ten-to-twelve-minute warmup, twenty-to-thirty-minute MEP, ten-to-twelve-minute cool-down. Total time: forty to fifty-four minutes.

Alternate Saturdays:

A MEP workout that starts at sixty minutes and increases in twenty-minute increments until you reach two hours; at that point, hold steady for two weeks.

Alternate Sundays:

A combo run/walk consisting of a fifteen-minute warmup walk, a fifteen-minute MAP run, a fifteen-minute walk, a fifteen-minute MEP run, a fifteen-minute walk, a fifteen-minute MAP run, and a fifteen-minute cool-down walk. Total time: one hour and forty-five minutes. (Every other week increase the run segments by ten minutes until reaching fifty-five minutes three weeks before the marathon, for a three-hour-and-forty-five-minute time commitment. The week before the marathon, the running segments are thirty minutes in length.)

Level Three: Up-Tempo, Challenging, and Vigorous

The main objective of level-three training is to provide your body with a wide assortment of training experiences in order to enhance physical performance, generate excitement, and increase the level of challenge in a controlled and systematic way. Once you have improved your fat-burning ability in level one and increased your efficiency in level two, you are ready for level three, which adds the weekly SAP speedy anaerobic pace challenges. In level three, you maintain a balance of peak fitness and optimal health by moving in all three cardio c-quences. The training is as simple as one, two, three. Each week you are scheduled to perform one SAP, two MEPs, and three MAPs, a 1:2:3 ratio. As in level two, training in level three will accelerate your productivity in the MEP zone. When implemented correctly, the proportion of one SAP to two MEPs to three MAPs blends rigorous, up-tempo challenges with productive and efficient workouts and comfortable, relaxing, and rejuvenating movement states.

Once you get into the level-three training program, you will notice how the flow of energy states takes on a natural rhythm all its own. You will start to look forward to each component of your training program. When the schedule calls for a calm and relaxing day, you will appreciate it because you know you will let loose later in the week. You will have the confidence that you are building a healthier and fitter future, while having fun and enjoying the process.

LEVEL-THREE CLIENT PROFILE

I am the director of the running program at New York's Chelsea Piers, where a regular group gathers for the Tuesday SAP workout. The group is comprised of the widest range imaginable, from absolute beginners to middle-aged weekend warrior businesspeople, to people like Amy, a 3:30 marathoner who's been running regularly for ten years. The SAP cardio c-quence routines are similar to the classic interval-style workout, where a short period of up-tempo effort is followed by a recovery period of the same or varying length. We start each SAP with a fifteen-minute walk, during which time the runners and I circle the track while I preview the workout. The warmup also serves as prime catching-up time, when all the participants can share training stories and life experiences with one another. At the end of the warmup walk, we begin our interval training. For the next thirty minutes, we divide the time equally between up-tempo SAP runs and recoveries in the MAP zone. I signify the start of each interval by blowing my whistle, which sets the runners off into their individual SAP cardio c-quences. With runners of such varied abilities circumnavigating the same track, the workout is quite a sight. The athletes circle the track, each one marching to the beat of his own heart-rate monitor. I blow the whistle a second time, and everyone winds down back into his or her MAP. Some people are walking; others jogging or running. There is so much excitement generated by the group. Part of it is due to the sharing of a common experience by such a diverse, talented crowd. I blow the whistle a third time and they're off and running—or fast-walking—once again.

Amy tells me this is her favorite workout. Prior to joining my running program, her interval training consisted of dreaded all-out sprints. She took each interval session like a good patient taking her medicine, hoping it would lead to improvement down the road.

The sessions were intensely competitive, she didn't have fun, and after a while her body started to hurt. The SAP workouts are different. They, too, are up-tempo and challenging but the focus is less on who can run the fastest and more on who can best manage her heart rate.

On Thursdays, I organize group MEP runs. We repeat the same fifteen-minute warmup, proceed into a thirty-minute MEP run, and finish with another fifteen-minute cool-down walk. Amy finds these workouts enjoyable and motivating, not draining and debilitating. In between our group sessions, I encourage her to do lots of MAP workouts and combo run/walks. On Saturdays, she repeats the MEP workout, extending it by thirty minutes every other Saturday when she is preparing for a performance event.

The point of balancing the MEPs with the MAPs and SAPs is to offer a range of experiences and fat- and sugar-burning states. Monitoring your pace in the MEP is the best indicator of whether the program is working. Through time you want your pace in the MEP to speed up. After two months in my running program, Amy flies out to do her second Los Angeles marathon. She finishes with the best marathon time she's had in ten years. She is ecstatic that she can have such an outstanding performance by letting go of her obsession with time and following her heart rate.

TYPICAL WEEK DURING TWELVE-WEEK TRAINING PROGRAM

Monday, Wednesday, Friday, Sunday:

Seven-to-ten-minute warmup, twenty-to-forty-five-minute MAP, seven-to-ten-minute cool-down, twenty minutes weights, five minutes abdominal workout. Total time: thirty-four to ninety minutes. MAP runs can be extended as long as the heart rate remains in target zone.

Tuesday:

Twelve-to-fifteen-minute warmup, SAP interval workout, twelve-to-fifteen-minute cool-down.

SAP INTERVAL WORKOUTS

Week one:

One-minute SAP followed by one-minute recovery in MAP repeated seven times.

Week two:

Three-minute SAP followed by three-minute recovery in MAP repeated three times.

Week three:

Ninety-second SAP followed by ninety-second recovery in MAP repeated five times.

Week four:

Five-minute SAP followed by three-minute recovery in MAP repeated two times.

Weeks five through eight:

Add one additional repeat to each SAP routine.

Weeks nine through twelve:

Add one additional repeat to each SAP routine.

Thursday and Saturday:

Ten-to-twelve-minute warmup, twenty-to-thirty-minute MEP, ten-to-twelve-minute cool-down. Total time: forty to fifty-four minutes.

Alternate Saturdays:

An MEP workout that starts at ninety minutes and increases in twenty-minute increments until you reach 2.5 hours on week eight. On week ten, drop back down to two hours.

Alternate Sundays:

Instead of the MAP, perform a combo run/walk consisting of a fifteen-minute warmup walk, followed by a twenty-minute MEP run, a fifteen-minute walk, a twenty-minute MEP run, a fifteen-minute walk, a twenty-minute MEP run, and a fifteen-minute cool-down walk. Total time: two hours. (Every other week increase the run segments by ten minutes until reaching three sixty-minute running segments three weeks before the marathon, for a final time commitment of four hours. The week before the marathon, the running segments return to thirty minutes in length.)

Now you understand my entire training program. The schedules outlined above demonstrate the potential that anyone can realize by running regularly. But the real indicator of success has nothing to do with running a marathon; it has to do with how movement enhances the quality of your life—no matter what your background or your goals.

I am reading a letter from Linda, a new client with five kids. As a stay-at-home mom, going to the gym every day isn't a reality. Instead, she's learned to incorporate movement into her daily routine. She walks laps around her house every morning. With a heart-rate monitor strapped to her chest, she rigorously does the chores. She is grateful for the newfound energy in her life. She realizes working out isn't just for professional athletes and beautiful people. It's a practice that can have a positive impact on everyone, even her.

Set your own running goals and break them down into daily and weekly routines. Maybe your goal is to run a marathon and you can follow one of the training schedules noted above. Or perhaps you, too, are just getting started and all you want to do is run around the block. Your training mustn't be tedious; make it fun and interesting. Share the experience with people you love. Or learn to the love new people with whom you train. Whatever your goals, the rewards are the absolute joy and the abundance of energy that comes from the ritual of running. Every day that you get out and move is a tremendous victory. Just move, as often as you can.

PART THREE

How to EAT for the Distance

No single aspect of "going the distance" triggers as much controversy as nutrition. I am tempted to include nutrition along with politics and religion as a topic that should not be discussed in public or among strangers. Eating isn't just something we do to meet our immediate nutrition and energy needs; it can be an emotionally charged statement of who we are and what we believe. My early memories of food involve weekend visits to my grandmother, who spent days joyously preparing meals for her children and grandchildren. Eating became an affirmation of our love for her. For some, food fills the void of a lonely moment, adding a modicum of joy and happiness when nothing else seems to work. For others, food is part of an epicurean celebration of life for which caution is thrown to the wind for the pleasure of the moment. It's an act of love between partners. A shared meal can be a communal experience, bringing families together and newcomers in the fold. Food choices are sometimes a social statement, such as the kind of vegetarianism born out of a desire not to kill animals or abstaining from eggs to keep baby chickens alive. The marketplace can also drive our day-to-day selection of food, using slick media campaigns that convince us a certain food or drink is essential when in reality it is not and may even be detrimental to our health and well-being.

On top of all this, exigencies of everyday life can influence whatever theories we may have about what to eat. Most of us do what it takes to get through the day, often eating on the run—literally. What results is a diet composed of foods that taste good, give quick bursts of energy, and are easy to purchase and prepare. Take a look at what most people eat and drink: pasta, bread, cereal, muffins, fast foods, energy bars and drinks, candy and cakes, soda, coffee, and alcohol—sugar, sugary foods, and dense, starchy carbohydrates that get converted by the body into sugar and trigger the release of insulin. The release of insulin not only destabilizes blood sugar and promotes fat storage but also leads to an insatiable appetite for more sugary foods. To make matters worse, the continued metabolism of sugar produces acid, ultimately making us lethargic and fatigued. In the long run, a reliance on carbohydrates and sugar undermines health, destabilizes energy, and diminishes your ability to go the distance. The simple truth is that energy from sugar creates a dependency on sugar. When we burn sugar we crave more sugar, compelling us to consume foods that satiate our body's growing dependency on sugar rather than its genuine nutritional needs.

So what's the way out? If you were to ask me, "What should I eat?" my initial response would be to find out more about who is asking the question. Effective coaching must emanate from an understanding of the client and world in which he or she lives. The coach must be sensitive and empathetic in order to be effective. An Arizona-based client who is a real-estate developer, going through a mid-life divorce, living on his own for the first time since college, is going to have a much different relationship to eating than the homemaker who lives on a farm in the Midwest with her husband and three children. Then there's the business executive in New York City whose life is lived on the go. The ritual of eating is as much about establishing contacts and generating business as it is about nutrition. If I were to suggest to him that he pull out a Tupperware bowl filled with mixed greens, tofu, and alfalfa sprouts while his associates dined on steak, wine, and crème brulée, his commitment to energetic eating might bring him greater health—but fewer clients. The executive wants to know what he can eat—at restaurants and at home—to maintain his energy for his hectic schedule. The homemaker wants to put together the healthiest meals for her and her family. The real-estate developer wants to learn how to eat in a way that will keep him youthful and extend his life.

So while there may be a few universal truths when it comes to nutrition—such as remove sugar from your diet, eat more vegetables, and drink plenty of water—the particular likes and dislikes, beliefs and personal rituals of each individual have to play a part in developing an energy-producing nutritional strategy. As you read through the information in this section and get to know the real-life stories of people who have changed their lives in substantial or in subtle ways, you'll eventually have to decide what level of commitment you want to make. Are you simply interested in fine-tuning your eating to get more energy or to reduce your weight? Maybe you're stuck right now because of conflicting information and you want to develop a plan that makes sense to you and move on. Perhaps a less-than-favorable report from your physician is the main impetus to review what you're doing and how you eat. Possibly you may be so committed to peak performance in the athletic arena or on the job that you will eagerly do whatever it takes to move on to the next level. Only you can answer these questions and choose the course of action that best suits you and the life you lead.

In any case, in order to get at the truth of what is best for you, you must first free yourself from food dependencies and careless habits. At some point I will make suggestions to wean yourself from sugar and get your body better at burning fat, which by now I hope I've succeeded in communicating to you is the best source of energy. Some of these recommendations will include steps that require you to cleanse and deacidify your body while removing from your diet those foods that make you dependent on sugar and inhibit your ability to burn fat. The ultimate goal is for you to reorganize your nutritional strategies around foods that get you burning fat, so you can optimize your health, stabilize your energy, and maximize your ability to go the distance. Once you are cleansed, balanced, and sugar-free, then and only then can you make great decisions about what foods to eat and how far you want to go in your journey toward nutritional excellence.

19

Generate Energy from Within

Early in my career my eating habits and nutrition strategies were fairly conventional, derived mostly from journals, popular running magazines, and whatever information I could coax from more experienced runners and coaches. By the time I entered competitive running in the late 1970s, I basically existed on a vegetarian version of the running culture diet. I ate tons of pasta, bread, and potatoes, with an occasional salad or steamed vegetable thrown in for good measure. Because of my high mileage, I believed it was not only acceptable but that I was entitled to treat myself to some Häagen Dazs or other sweet indulgence for dessert. Like most other aspiring competitive runners, I consumed as little fat as possible in order to try to keep my weight down and my body fat low. Besides, almost everything I read or heard from other runners proclaimed that fat, either in my food or in my body, would slow me down. I came to believe that carbs and carbs alone were a runner's best friend. The legendary running guru of the 1970s, Jim Fixx, in his famous work *The Complete Book of Running*, encouraged runners to lean more toward carbohydrates than fats. He reinforced the point by describing how a well-known coach prepared for an ultramarathon by loading up on raisin cookies. The story was similar to others I was aware of, so for the next six years I thrived on a carbohydrate-rich diet while I radically increased my miles, running as many as thirty miles a day.

By the summer of 1982, I was a professional endurance athlete, a consultant to Nike, and the national spokesman for Gatorade. I went on to set my third consecutive American record for the hundred-mile race and, one year later, a new American record in a six-day run broadcast nationally by Ted Koppel and the ABC News program *Nightline*. Later that same year, I entered the Ironman World Triathlon Championship in Kona, Hawaii, and ended up seventy-third out of a thousand race participants. Even more incredibly, I finished second in the celebrated double Ironman called Ultraman three months later. I was now entering a new phase of my career that placed me among the top endurance athletes in the world. Yet underneath all these accomplishments was a body that was beginning to betray me.

Even though I was fairly successful, I was not feeling that great. Throughout most of the previous year, my body had begun to show signs of wear and tear. By the spring of 1984, I entered my second six-day race, and by then my right foot, in particular, was bothering me. I struggled mightily during the event and barely managed to come in a disappointing seventh place. Searching for reasons, I could only conclude that my breakdown was the inevitable outcome of running as many miles as I did. I did not, even for a moment, consider that my diet might have something to do with how I felt. I had been operating under the assumption that my nutritional standards were fairly high. After all, I made a tremendous effort to watch my diet. As is the habit with most ultrarunners, during a race I relied heavily on carbohydrate-rich foods such as potatoes, bread, cookies, peanut butter and jelly sandwiches, and sports drinks. I signed on to the prevailing running culture notion that the more carbs I ate, the more energy I'd have. My conception of food was no different than an engineer on an old steam locomotive; all I was doing was shoveling coal into a furnace to create the steam necessary to drive the train.

One month before I was scheduled to travel to France for my next big race, I met the now-famous Dr. Phil Maffetone at a triathlon and discussed my plight with him. He worked on me and convinced me to get sugar out of my diet, eat more oils, and dramatically increase my consumption of water. Just one month after my forgettable seventh-place finish, I was back competing, setting another American record for the six-day race with 571 miles. I was able to run a remarkable 70 miles more than my previous best of 501.

The encounter with Maffetone became even more extraordinary for other reasons. As I mentioned earlier, probably the most important outcome of our initial time working together was getting to recognize the importance burning fat has on endurance and health. Equally important and inextricably intertwined with the burning of fat was Phil's contention that "you need to eat fat in order to burn fat." My world was beginning to turn upside down. Fat, the nutrient that I had been avoiding for years, was now being championed as the key ingredient that ignites the body's fat-burning system. This new worldview blamed starchy and concentrated carbohydrates for inhibiting fat utilization and promoting sugar-burning and fat storage.

Challenging myself to let go of everything I believed to be true and trying out an alternative approach to nutrition wasn't easy. However, I was so intrigued with the concept of burning fat and overjoyed with the results I was getting that I stuck with my new food program. I continued to abstain from eating most carbohydrate-based, sugar-laden foods such as pasta, breads, cakes, cookies, and fruit. In their place I ate plenty of fresh vegetables and fish, with only a moderate reliance on grains such as rice and quinoa. I started using extra-virgin olive oil mixed with the juice of freshly squeezed lemons and chopped garlic on my salads, ate more fish and occasionally some organic meat, and took one teaspoon of cold-pressed flaxseed oil with meals. In May of 1986, all of my efforts came to fruition as I set a new standard by running a thousand miles in a world record eleven days and twenty hours.

I am circling the track after many days of running and becoming acutely aware that my relationship to eating is gradually transforming. When I first started competing in multiday events, I viewed meal breaks as a welcome relief from an otherwise tedious and austere day. Food is instant gratification in a world devoid of pleasure; it exists only to provide me with immediate energy and pleasure and enough of an incentive to keep me going until my next meal break. Now, after changing my nutrition strategies to rely more on a balanced approach to eating, not just on carbohydrates for energy, I've come to recognize that moving itself is what I crave—not the eating. I feel as if I can move continuously, effortlessly, and forever. Food is now the means to an end, not an end in and of itself. Meal breaks are no longer a welcome relief from the austere and tiring act of running; they provide the ingredients that release the energy I have stored within me. In essence, my relationship to food has flipped-flopped. Eating is no longer the reward for continuously moving; being able to continuously move is the reward for eating right.

The meals themselves become smaller and more numerous. I notice I am always full of energy and never hungry. I no longer evaluate the success of my meals by how much immediate energy they give me. My conception of palatability is changing dramatically. The more simply prepared, less sweetened, and natural the food tastes, the more stable and dependable my energy feels. Conversely, the sweeter and more processed the food tastes, the more unstable and undependable my energy feels. Now, as I am eating, I recognize that the true value of the meal comes later, when I experience how sustainable and everlasting my energy becomes. I experience a sense of priming a fat-burning pump rather than recharging a dead battery. The feeling I have now is so far removed from the one I once got from a cup of coffee or cookie. It is much more even and durable, and it lasts for a noticeably longer periods, with fewer highs and lows. In this state of motion, I am always in control and have the power to make myself feel good. It is an eating style and attitude that I am committed to integrating into my day-to-day life.

20

Change Your Diet, Change Your Life

Almost immediately after the thousand-mile race, I suspended my competitive schedule and resumed my graduate studies in exercise physiology at Columbia University. I wanted to systematically evaluate my training methods so I could formulate a program that others could follow. I began educating myself about the role training and nutrition play in influencing energy metabolism, and from what source—fat or sugar—we get our energy. My research led me to examine the role insulin plays in energy metabolism.

Insulin plays a significant role in sugar usage and the fat storage. How effectively insulin performs depends on how much aerobic, fat-burning exercise you get (aerobic exercise makes you more sensitive to insulin) and by what you eat. Normally, the carbohydrates you eat get converted to sugar. As sugar levels rise, insulin is secreted by the pancreas to transport sugar into the cells to be used as fuel (energy). During optimal conditions, insulin production is limited to the amount needed to stimulate the metabolism of the ingested carbohydrates (sugars). However, the excessive consumption of carbohydrates can throw off this delicate and precise dynamic between insulin and blood sugar and lead to too much insulin production.

I recommend that most people eat only small amounts of grains, baked goods, and pastas because many people have trouble processing these dense, starchy carbohydrates. Have you ever had a muffin or bagel for breakfast, and by 10:00 A.M. you're in need of caffeine or another "hit" of something sweet to wake you up? A noticeable drop in energy after the initial high of eating a carbohydrate-laden meal could be an indication that you are somewhat carbohydrate intolerant. Carbohydrate Intolerance (CI) is a phenomenon spoken of by many researchers, including Dr. Barry Sears, author of *The Zone,* and Dr. Phil Maffetone. They both speculate that an extensive number of people tend toward carbohydrate intolerance.

How can so many people have trouble ingesting carbohydrates? CI logic is based on the fact that the bulk of human evolution occurred prior to the introduction of large amounts of carbohydrates into the food chain. The human digestive systems evolved on a diet of lean meats, vegetables, and fruits. Not until the advent of agriculture, somewhere between ten thousand and thirty thousand years ago, were significant amounts of grains and dairy products introduced. Many people have difficulty processing these nutrients, especially in a concentrated form: e.g., pastas, baked goods, grains, cereals, milk, and ice cream.

A person with carbohydrate intolerance has difficulty in processing carbohydrates and through time must secrete more and more insulin to break down the carbohydrates into sugar and carry it into the cells for energy. As insulin gets secreted in higher and higher doses, it sweeps sugar out of the blood and into the cells, causing blood-sugar levels to drop. The drop in blood-sugar level triggers a craving for more sugar, so additional carbohydrates must be consumed. If you succumb to this craving, you stimulate more insulin secretion and another drop in blood sugar, which in turn provokes more sugar cravings, sugar consumption, and ultimately another rise in insulin secretion, and so on.

Thus, the carbohydrate-intolerant individual tends to have elevated insulin levels and can get caught up in the vicious circle of carbohydrate ingestion followed by energy lows followed by carbohydrate cravings, leading to carbohydrate ingestion and a repeat of the pattern. Symptoms of carbohydrate intolerance include drowsiness after high-carbohydrate meals, spells of poor concentration, feeling bloated after meals, creeping levels of fat around your waist, and gradual rises in blood pressure, serum cholesterol, and triglycerides. The overabundance of insulin caused by CI and an excessive amount of carbohydrates in the diet can make the body less responsive to insulin secretions, and cause a more serious condition called hyperinsulemia. Hyperinsulemia (elevated blood-insulin levels) is a condition linked with diabetes, heart disease, and certain forms of cancer.

While the causes of carbohydrate intolerance and hyperinsulemia are not clear, almost everyone agrees that both genes and lifestyle are likely influences. Richard and Rachael Heller, in *The Carbohydrate Addict's Diet*, describe a process whereby the ingestion of large amounts of carbohydrates desensitizes the body's response to insulin and triggers ever larger secretions of insulin. As insulin levels rise dramatically, levels of serotonin—a neurotransmitter that is linked to appetite suppression—lag behind. This imbalance between insulin and serotonin renders serotonin ineffectual in producing a sense of appetite satisfaction. In other words, you're always hungry for carbs.

While insulin is a necessary chemical that breaks down sugar and carries it into the cells to be burned for energy, having too much insulin is not good. In fact, an excessive amount of insulin is the enemy of enduring energy and fat-burning. To make matters even worse, when you're in this sugar-burning/sugar-craving state, insulin also assumes the role of fat "maker." As you consume more carbohydrates to satiate sugar cravings, whatever sugar cannot be used or stored (there is little storage space for excess sugar) is converted into fat by insulin and deposited in the copious and expandable fat vaults located throughout the body.

The bottom line is that keeping your insulin level low is crucial. This means avoiding foods that are high-glycemic, or rapid inducers of insulin. High-glycemic foods, which are quickly converted by the body into sugar and stimulate a large and rapid insulin release, include all refined and simple sugars, cakes and candies, and even what may at first seem to be good food choices such as corn flakes, French bread, oat bran, rice cakes, carrots, bananas, red and yellow vegetables, and low-fat ice cream. On the other hand, foods such as green leafy vegetables, whole-grain rye bread, apples, black-eyed peas, and plums are low glycemic. Low-glycemic foods break down into sugar at a much slower rate and induce a much more gradual release of insulin. Somewhere in between are foods that stimulate the secretion of insulin at a moderate rate: oranges, garbanzo beans, high-fat potato chips, and peas. You can combine moderate- and high-glycemic foods with a healthy oil or fat or a protein to slow down the rate at which they are converted to sugar and make them act more like a low-glycemic food. For instance, a rice cake, an extremely high-glycemic food, can be transformed into a much slower inducer of insulin by topping it with nut butter, such as almond or macadamia nuts, which contain both healthy fatty oil and protein.

When you consume high-glycemic food, insulin levels rise dramatically and ultimately destabilize blood sugar by sweeping it out of the blood and into the cells. This drop in blood sugar—called hypoglycemia—leads to low energy and an ensuing craving for carbohydrates and sugary foods. Protect yourself by eating low-glycemic foods or combining higher glycemic foods with a healthy oil or protein-rich food. When your insulin levels are low and your blood sugar is stable, you can maintain constant and enduring energy levels and ensure that your fat usage will be high.

When I came to realize the dangers of high-glycemic foods and excessive insulin production, I decided to change my eating habits and include more high-quality fat in my meals. I was completely over any "fat-phobia" that might have lingered from my early running days. I was ready for the insulin-curtailing, burn-fat-promoting eating strategy that foreshadowed the 40:30:30 carbohydrate-to-fat-to-protein ratio that Sears later extolled in *The Zone*.

Little by little, my diet has continued to evolve. I never eat a carbohydrate by itself, build all my meals around protein, and consider the consequences of what I eat on insulin secretion. I drizzle olive oil over my salads and enjoy a wide variety of fish, an occasional egg, and even an infrequent piece of red meat or free-range organic chicken. Now, having studied it and lived it, I am ready to share this message with others.

When you think about it, the endurance athlete's mission to be as productive as possible for as long as possible is not much different from the mission most people face every day. Every week I counsel clients on eating strategies that will help them to unleash their innate energy so they remain strong and positive over the course of a challenging day—and then have the capability to get up the next day and do it again and again; endlessly and forever.

The Story of Ed, the Sugar Burner

Ed, like all of my clients, is a most remarkable individual. A city councilman, attorney, husband, and fitness enthusiast, he maintains a schedule that impresses even a multiday running specialist like myself. Because of his time challenges, he never keeps a regular routine. Over the course of a week, though, he is always able to squeeze in three to four workouts in my training facility even though he seems to be worn out when he arrives. He rushes in to the gym, changes, entrances my staff and me with stories of government and law as he dutifully slogs through another workout with one of my trainers. When his workout is done, he quickly showers and then is off to his next appointment in the blink of an eye.

One day, after a particularly comatose training session, Ed leaves his trainer, approaches me, and confesses that while he enjoys coming to the gym, he doesn't feel his energy level changing. While he is able to push himself through the course of his hectic appointment schedule, he finds himself at the brink of exhaustion by the time he gets home, which isn't exactly enhancing his relationship with his wife. He asks me what more he can do, besides his physical training, to increase his energy. I already know a bit about Ed and his lifestyle, so I ask him tell me what he eats. I've become so sensitive to this issue because I've experienced first-hand how the choice of foods can impact on the quality and consistency of the energy we create.

"What do you eat for breakfast?" I ask him. He sheepishly confesses that he usually doesn't eat anything at all until later in the day. He's tried eating in the morning, but found it only made him ravenously hungry by mid-morning. So he stopped eating breakfast and found he could make it to lunch without eating anything at all. The only problem was that by then he felt famished and unfocused. I know from experience that this is the moment when we are all the most susceptible to making poor food choices. For Ed, this usually means loading up on bread while waiting for his lunch to arrive, usually a sandwich, some chips, a cup of coffee, and dessert. It wasn't long before whatever surge of energy he felt from eating lunch began to wane, leaving him drowsy, unable to concentrate, and ravenously hungry. Ed's only remedy was to hit the vending machines for a granola bar and a soda.

I then ask Ed what he eats on the mornings that he does have breakfast. He replies, "You know, the typical stuff. A muffin or bagel, but only low-fat muffins and low-fat cream cheese on my bagel. Sometimes I'll have a breakfast bar in the car." Here's the part Ed can't figure out: Whether he does have breakfast or he doesn't have breakfast, he's always exhausted at the end of the day.

"Ed, I think I know what's going on here," I tell him. "You're relying on sugar for energy. The muffins, bagels, and the breakfast bars are all turned into sugar by the body. All you're doing throughout the day is feeding your body sugar so it's burning sugar. Compounding the issue, each time you eat one of these foods you're getting a massive hit of insulin, which sweeps sugar out of your blood, creating a sugar low that you can only rectify by eating more of the same food. No wonder you're hungry all day long! Your strategy may help you through the short-term, but over the period of days and weeks the consistency of your energy will suffer."

In an attempt to better understand how dependent Ed has become on carbohydrates as an energy source, I decide to take his waist-to-hip measurement (see instructions on page 229.) The waist-to-hip ratio compares the size of a person's waist to the size of his or her hips. It is based on the observation that the more carbohydrate-dependent a person becomes, the more apt he or she is to store fat in the midsection—a sign that a person is becoming dependent on carbohydrates. This midsection bulge results from the body's inability to process carbohydrates in the first place. The body's challenge with the carbohydrates leads to the oversecretion on insulin. It's the insulin that then takes the sugar out of the blood and stores it as fat, leaving the blood lacking in sugar and the person ravenously craving more carbohydrates. For men, a waist-to-hip ratio above 0.9 is reflective of a high dependency on sugar as an energy source and has been associated with an increased incidence of hyperinsulemia, high blood pressure, and diabetes. (The figure for women is 0.8.) Ed's waist-to-hip ratio turns out to be 38/36 or 1.03.

Ed is eager to know what he can do to break the sugar-dependency cycle. He wants me to tell him what he can eat in the morning that will sustain his energy throughout his frenetic day. Before I do, I want to make sure he understands a key point. "The energy that food can provide you is in no way comparable to the energy your body can release," I explain. "The same fuel that empowered me to run a thousand miles can empower you to maximize what you do as you participate in the thousand-mile race of your life, no matter how hectic and unrelenting it may seem. That fuel comes from within you, not from outside of you. The fat already stored in your body, not food, is your most enduring and reliable source of energy. Like an endurance athlete, you must learn to think of your food strategies as a means to release your own vast energy supply, which is stored body fat, rather than depend on food as fuel that eventually gets burned.

"You must never let your body become so depleted of energy that you begin to believe that the only way to revitalize yourself is by eating foods that give you a burst of energy. If you let yourself get into this pattern of pushing yourself to the brink of exhaustion and using food to resurrect your energy, eating takes on a meaning that goes beyond keeping you nourished and moves you into the realm of reactive urgency. You do not want to get caught in a repetitive cycle in which you run out of gas and your only option is to fill up the tank up by eating. In this energy-needy state, it's easy to fall into the trap of eating only those foods that give you an immediate surge, which are carbohydrate-based, sugar-rich foods, and flash-in-the-pan energizers such as coffee and soda.

"Get-energy-quick schemes force you to rely on exogenous energy sources in the form of carbohydrates and sugary foods and drinks. While offering a quick burst of energy, these carbohydrate-dependent strategies direct you away from your body's inherent energy and entrap you into a reliance on sugar. In effect, by eating large of amounts of carbohydrates, you block the pathway to your body's energy stores, which prevents you from accessing your nearly infinite reserves of fat. You may experience a noticeable and immediate energy 'high' from ingesting sugar-based foods, but it is short-lived and almost always followed by a energy 'low,' which can only be uplifted by another hit of sugar. This alternation sets in motion a continuous, up-and-down cycle that is strung together by repeated doses of sugar ingestion and sugar cravings.

"The way out of the cycle is to shift your thinking and your diet. Again, you never want to get into an energy-needy state in the first place, which happens when you draw energy from the small fuel tank that is filled with sugar. The most powerful and dependable eating strategies steer you to the fat-filled fuel tank that can't be emptied. The way you draw from this energy-abundant 'big' tank is to minimize your consumption of insulin-inducing, sugar-laden, carbohydrate-rich meals devoid of fat, which destabilize your energy level and weaken you in the long run. Start by eliminating dense, starchy, and wheat-based carbs, such as muffins, bagels, cakes, breads, potatoes, and pasta. Replace them with low-glycemic foods such as green vegetables, fish, seeds, nuts, and plenty of water and high quality essential fats such as olive, linseed (flax), and fish oil. You can supplement these foods with higher-glycemic choices such as rice, beans, sweet potatoes, carrots, and turnips as long as you remember to combine them with healthy oils such as olive oil or flaxseed oil and proteins such as fish, seeds, and nuts and nut butters.

"This strategy will keep your insulin levels low, blood sugar stable, and encourage your body to access its own fat stores. By doing so, you, like the successful endurance athlete, can meet your primary objective, which is to create consistent, long-lasting, health-promoting energy that comes from fat. In the fat-burning mode, you will possess the enduring energy and vitality to get moving and keep moving all hours of the day.

"One final way to ensure you stay on this energy-rich path is to borrow from the performance strategy of a multiday specialist, who never lets himself get to the point where he's too tired to go anymore and is forced to break out of necessity. The endurance athlete remains in control by preemptively scheduling regular breaks. Apply this lesson to your eating strategy by organizing small eating breaks spread evenly throughout the day so that you never let yourself become famished and in dire need of food."

Ed looks at me quizzically, and I remember that he is close to his brother-in-law, who is a medical doctor. They share a fairly traditional point of view on nutrition: Try not to eat too much and get regular exercise. The idea that certain eating strategies have life-changing capabilities is not part of Ed's global view. I know with Ed that if I were to suggest he go to a health-food store, he'd roll his eyes, mockingly give me a peace sign, and ask me to think of something else. Finally, he says he's open to change within reason, though he still doesn't understand from where he'll get his energy if he gives up carbohydrates. "It'll come from your body," I tell him. "But don't just depend on me. Trust your body." I ask him to commit for one week to see how he feels, and he agrees.

"We don't have to make the changes so dramatic," I tell him. "But you do need to stop eating sugar and baked goods for a week to break you from you dependency on sugar." For breakfast, instead of muffins or a bagel, I recommend he has a salad, a plate full of sliced cucumbers and broccoli, or some steamed vegetables. Add to these vegetables a little bit of rice and a small piece of salmon that you prepare the night before, and lightly cover everything with olive oil and fresh squeezed lemon juice. What I'd really like him to do is start each day with a vegetable drink made of spinach, kale, cucumbers, fresh parsley, garlic, celery, and fresh ginger in the morning or a powdered vegetable drink comprised of a blend of natural grasses and sprouted grains called Super Greens. When I bring it up, he says he'll think about it. I say, "If I make it for you, will you drink it?" He agrees, and in the meantime commits to reduce his coffee intake from six cups a day to two cups of decaf. For lunch, he can eat a large salad sprinkled with any of the following items: water-soaked pumpkin and sunflower seeds and almonds, tofu, tuna, sardines, or sliced eggs. He can add to his meals a fat-burning salad dressing made of three parts olive oil to one part fresh lemon juice (no vinegar) seasoned with freshly minced garlic or a seasoning called Mrs. Dash or Bragg's Aminos. Dinner can be fresh fish lightly drizzled with olive oil, steamed vegetables, and another salad. For one entire week he must commit to no sugary desserts or fruits. He can snack on almonds, seeds, celery stalks smeared with almond butter, or have an extra salad or some more steamed vegetables with olive oil, lemon, and fresh garlic. "You must keep reminding yourself that this will be for one week and you may actually begin to feel great," I tell him.

He asks whether he can eat beef or poultry. My response is that I prefer he eat these instead of the starchy carbohydrates he has been eating. I request, however, that should he choose to eat beef or poultry, it be of the highest quality possible— preferably organic, free-range, or kosher. My main concern is getting him off of sugar and dense carbohydrates first and we'll build from there.

After only a few days, Ed experiences a noticeable increase in energy. This gives him the leverage to maintain his new eating habits, as odd as they may seem, for the entire seven days. At the end of the weeklong trial period, Ed is willing to continue with certain aspects of his nutrition plan, though he still isn't comfortable radically changing his diet right at the moment. For breakfast, the idea of waking up and eating a green salad doesn't appeal to him, even though he now sees the benefits of minimizing sugar and carbohydrates in his diet. He agrees to cut out bagels, muffins, and low-fat breakfast bars and replace them with rice cakes and almond butter or two eggs on whole grain rye bread or Rye Vita crackers. I tell him that soups are excellent sources of nourishment throughout the day, as long as he avoids cream-based ones and those that contain noodles and other forms of pasta. Recommended soups are vegetable soup, tomato soup, chicken and rice, lentil soup, split pea, and bean soups with a salad instead of a roll. It is my turn to confess to Ed that I privately attribute my success during the later stages of my multiday running career to my mom's vegetable soup.

As a city councilman, Ed goes to a lot of dinners. He learns to ask for extra sides of vegetables instead of potatoes or pasta. He orders his salads without any dressing and requests olive oil, lemon wedges, and freshly minced garlic on the side to make his own salad dressing. He sticks to simply prepared fish, chicken, and occasionally some red meat, which he doesn't want to give up. He makes a habit of asking waiters to remove the bread from the table so it's not there to tempt him. He does the best he can to drink water throughout the day so when he sits down to his meals he's not thirsty. Alcohol, which is high-glycemic, he limits to one or two glasses of wine with dinner, and he is willing to give up his scotch.

By letting go of high-glycemic foods and high-glycemic eating habits, Ed has seen a lot of positive changes in his life. He now eats sensibly throughout the day instead of waiting until he's starving—a practice that gives him more consistent energy. He needs only six hours of sleep a night instead of his usual seven or eight and has more enthusiasm for doing things in the evening with his wife.

Old Nutrition Plan
(ENERGY-DRAINING MEALS)

New Nutrition Plan
(ENERGY-GENERATING MEALS)

Breakfasts:

cup of coffee with milk and sugar
bagel with low-fat cream cheese

Breakfasts:

green vegetable drink
two eggs fried in butter served on 100
percent whole-grain rye

rice cakes with almond butter
vegetable soup
green salad and plate of cucumbers
   with olive oil and lemon dressing
sautéed vegetables with salmon and
   jasmine rice

Snacks:

breakfast bar
granola bar
fruit pop tarts
coffee

Snacks:

almonds soaked in water overnight
pumpkin seeds
celery sticks with almond butter
sliced cucumbers with olive oil,
   lemon, and garlic dip

Lunches:

chicken-salad sandwich and chips
slice of pizza
corned beef sandwich with sauerkraut

Lunches:

big mixed green salad with sardines
   or tuna, nuts, and fat-burning salad
   dressing
soup and salad (no bread)
sprouted-wheat tortilla filled with
   steamed vegetables sautéed in olive oil

Dinners:

steak, potatoes, vegetables,
   and small salad

dessert—cake, pie, or ice cream

Dinners:

steamed vegetables with simply prepared grilled fish and a small serving
   of rice
stir-fry vegetables with roasted lamb
sushi
sautéed spinach with red snapper
romaine salad with feta cheese,
   onions, red pepper, and sardines

Beverages:	Beverages:
4 to 6 cups of regular coffee or latte with sugar, juice, iced tea, sports drinks, and cocktails	1 to 2 cups of decaffeinated coffee with milk, no sugar constantly sipping on two to three liters of water a day 3 to 5 cups of green vegetable drink, 4 to 6 glasses of wine per week

Ed is learning to examine and experiment with his dietary options to make himself so in tune with his body that he will be able to follow it wherever it wants to go. He reminds me of so many of my clients who are comfortable within the boundaries that they have already set but are moving toward the edge, ready for a change. As a coach I want to support Ed as he steps beyond the familiar and begins to explore the possibilities of what might be. Sometimes, I have to remind myself that the smallest of changes can still lead to the most powerful results. If I hold him up to an absolute standard so far removed from his customary experience, I will probably set him up to fail. Instead, I preferred to create a series of realizable goals for Ed that he can attain every day, building on his daily successes. I want Ed to wake up every morning and ask himself, "Is there one more thing I can do differently today than yesterday that will lead me to unbounded energy?"

THE WAIST-TO-HIP TEST:
WAIST DIVIDED BY HIPS = WAIST-TO-HIP RATIO

Monitoring your waist-to-hip ratio is a great way to assess whether your nutritional strategies are moving you toward or away from a dependency on carbohydrates. The waist-to-hip ratio is derived by measuring the circumference of the waist just above the naval and dividing that number by the measurement of the widest region around the hips. High waist-to-hip ratios above 0.8 for women and 0.9 for men are associated with higher rates of hyperinsulemia, high trygliceride levels, high blood pressure and insulin-resistant (Type II) diabetes. These symptoms develop as a result of sugar-burning, fat-storing eating habits. Carbohydrate-intolerant, insulin-resistant individuals tend to deposit fat in the waist area.

Determining your waist-to-hip ratio is easy; all you need is a tape measure and a calculator. I recommend you take the measurements without your clothes on to ensure the readings are accurate and reliable over time. However, you may take them with your clothes on as long as you remember to do it exactly the same next time you take the measurement.

Step 1:

Using a cloth measuring tape, measure the circumference of your waist approximately one inch above your naval. Pull the tape measure snugly, but not too tight. For best results, get a partner and take the measurement from the side of your waist as opposed to the front or back.

Step 2:

Repeat the process, using the same technique for your hip measurement, which is the widest circumference of your body around the hip and buttock area. Use your best judgement to gauge where that will be. Position the tape so that it crosses over the fleshiest part of the buttocks, parallel to the ground.

Step 3:

Divide your waist measure by your hip measure. For example, a woman with waist measurement of 29 inches and a hip measurement of 36 inches would calculate her waist-to-hip ratio as follows: 29 divided by 36 equals 0.80.

A man with a waist of 32 and a hip measure of 36 would have a waist-to-hip ratio of .88.

If your measurements are right around or below .8 for women and .9 for men, you are probably not depending on sugar as an energy source and are fairly good at burning fat. If your waist-to-hip ratio is above these values, you might want to decrease the amount of sugar and sugar-based foods in your diet.

You can check your waist-to-hip ratio at the beginning and at the end of your seven-to-ten-day cleanse and on a regular basis thereafter—minimally every three months and no more than every two or three weeks.

21

Make Friends with Fat

There's a simple, humbling truth in the notion that all nutrients are good as long as their presence in your life reflects the natural order of the world and the reality of your own personal existence. Even the most dreaded of all fats—saturated fats—can have a place in the human diet. The by-products of saturated fat work in combination with other types of fats and are absolutely essential in the healing process. The question of whether humans should or should not ingest *any* food containing saturated fat is a discussion that is best carried on by someone else in some other context. As your coach, I'm less interested in convincing you that one nutritional doctrine is superior to another than in inspiring you to make the first step toward reorganizing your current food strategies so they work even better for you. I am comfortable with the notion that saturated fats exist for a reason, and the goal is to achieve an optimal balance between them and the other fats in your diet so you always move in a direction in which you're burning fat and enjoying enduring energy and optimal health.

When I hear someone say that a food has fat in it, it means something totally different to me than it did fifteen years ago. Whereas once it meant that a particular food should be avoided, now I view fat as something that is indispensable to my diet. The main questions I want to answer are what type of fat is it and how much of it do I want.

A growing number of researchers, coaches, and endurance enthusiasts recognize the role that fats play in maintaining consistent energy over the long run. Fats have twice as many calories per unit as do carbohydrates and protein, making them the highest concentration of energy on the planet. I promise that if you're in the middle of an endurance event looking for compact yet potent sources of power, this is a very attractive concept. Yet what really matters is not so much that the fat has energy in it but that the ingestion of fat makes it more likely that your body will tap into and burn the fat it already has.

Still, for all their value, in popular culture fats remain taboo. In a society where health and fitness are reduced to "weight management," "getting thin," and "running a faster time," fats have become a stigma. For one, they're calorically dense. When people are trying to lose weight and fat, they are taught that the higher caloric value of fats make them something to be avoided rather than something to include. People then try to eat less fat so they can continue eating more food. This kind of thinking makes you vulnerable to marketing campaigns that extol the benefits of fat-free and low-fat foods and fat substitutes. While these foods may be low in fat, they are rich in sugar and can promote the massive release of insulin, which can have far worse implications on your energy and health.

Secondly, implicit in the message that eating fats will make us fat is the warning that consuming too much fat is a health risk. We have all heard plenty about the link between excess dietary fats and the increased risk of heart disease and cancer, often with regard to cholesterol, a type of fat only found in animals. Advertising campaigns launched by margarine and cereal companies warn us of the dangers associated with foods containing cholesterol so that we won't eat eggs but rather their own brand of egg-substitutes. Dairy manufacturers get into the act by coming out with entire lines of fat-free and low-fat milk and milk products such as cheese, yogurt, and ice cream. Is it any wonder so many people are scared to eat anything with fat or cholesterol in it?

The truth is that the ingestion of fat is essential to human life. All of our cells are coated with a biolipid (fatty) layer that maintains and protects the integrity of each individual cell. Fats protect the hair and skin from external pollutants and give it luster and shine from within. Without dietary fat, the human body cannot absorb fat-soluble vitamins such as A, D, E, and K and calcium, the mineral essential for maintaining bone density. Vitamin D itself is a derivative of the interaction of sunlight with cholesterol found in the skin. The vitamin D formed by the exposure of cholesterol in our bodies to sunlight gets absorbed into the blood, which then allows calcium and phosphorus to be absorbed from the intestinal tract. Once assimilated into the blood, prostaglandin, a hormonelike chemical that is also a derivative of dietary fat, must then be available in order to carry calcium into the bones. Besides facilitating the absorption of calcium, other kinds of dietary fat-derived prostaglandins participate in a vast array of cellular functions, including controlling inflammation, maintaining proper hydration, promoting blood circulation, fighting bacterial and viral infection, and regulating free radical production.

Fats and fat derivatives are responsible for a wide variety of hormonal responses. For instance, the adrenal glands rely on cholesterol to produce progesterone, which is necessary to promote healthy female sexual function, reproduction, and fetal growth. Cholesterol is also used by the adrenals to produce cortisone, which helps to ease the pain of normal inflammation in the muscles and bones after you exercise or perform a physically challenging act.

Fats from your diet aid digestion. The presence of fats in the diet enables the liver to secrete bile, which your small intestine needs in order to digest fats. The presence of fats in the diet also slows down the rate at which food gets emptied out of the stomach. Many people—runners in particular—believe that they want food to pass through their digestive systems as quickly as possible. Runners are tempted to think that the more energy the body has to expend digesting a meal, the less time and energy it will have for running. Or they reason that the faster food passes through the digestive system, the "lighter" they will feel and the faster they can run. Applying this logic, it would seem that slowing down the rate at which food passes through the digestive system is *not* a good thing. Yet it is! By slowing down the rate of passage, the body has a greater chance to absorb the nutrients from the foods you eat. And the presence of fat in the diet slows down the rate at which sugar is absorbed in the small intestines, keeping insulin secretions low and the opportunity to burn fat high.

Fats protect us from harm. The layer of fat in Eskimos guards them against the severe cold and otherwise uninhabitable Arctic conditions. The layer of fats around the cells seems to safeguard us from the insidious and omnipresent danger of radiation, from the sun, from airplane flights, and from x-rays.

One final word about fat before we move on. Meals with fat in them taste better. The chances are much greater that you will be satisfied—and actually eat less—if the foods you eat contain fats. As we stated earlier, if foods don't contain fats, they will contain more of something else, most likely carbohydrates that the body converts into sugar. Once again, and this bears repeating, fat-free and low-fat foods are by definition sugar-rich. The combination of low-fat/sugar-rich can only leave you hungry and dissatisfied and dependent on sugar and sugar substitutes to add delectability to a product that has been made bland-tasting by having the flavorful fat removed.

With dietary fat serving so many vital functions, it is a wonder that fat has become the enemy and sugar-rich, low-fat, no-fat, and cholesterol-free products have turned up in its place. Yet, ironically, some of the very products claiming to be "healthy" fat alternatives have recently been associated with an increased risk of heart disease and cancer. Researchers at Harvard University and the University of North Carolina linked the consumption of high levels of trans-fatty acids—found in margarine, baked goods, and processed foods, among other products—to a greater risk of heart disease and breast cancer. A trans-fatty acid is usually made from a vegetable oil—corn, cottonseed, or soybean, for example—that has been treated by a process called hydrogenation to make it a solid at room temperature.

When margarine first appeared in the marketplace, consumers were led to believe they could lower their risk of heart disease and cancer by using this product. All they had to do was replace products containing saturated fat—such as butter, chicken fat, and lard, which had been linked to increased risk of heart disease and cancer—with this new vegetable-based product made of polyunsaturated oil. What later became evident is that the chemical process that made vegetable oil "look" like a saturated fat by solidifying at room temperature caused it to act like one as well, making high levels of either fat a health risk.

One particularly insidious aspect of trans-fatty acids is that they alter the normal metabolism of fats by creating a deficiency of the fatty acids necessary to burn fat. In other words, unlike a natural fat, which will promote the utilization of fat as an energy source, trans-fatty acids do the opposite, causing you to store fat and burn sugar. Trans-fatty acids may also actually increase the levels of low-density lipoproteins (LDL), or "bad" cholesterol, while decreasing high-density lipoproteins (HDL), or "good" cholesterol, in your body—not the effect you want!

Shun all foods containing trans-fatty oils. Eating them is not worth the risk. Identifying foods that contain these potentially dangerous oils is not that difficult. As a general rule, trans-fatty oils can be found in foods that have to sit on a shelf, such as baked goods, snack chips, some national brands of peanut butter, candy bars, cookies, and the like. Before you purchase a food, check the ingredients to see if it contains "partially hydrogenated oils," the term used to identify trans-fatty acids. Terming these hydro-genated trans-fatty acids "partially hydrogenated oils" reminds me of the phrase "sort of pregnant." Consider the oil either hydro-genated or not. If the label lists "partially hydrogenated oil" as an ingredient, find a substitute that contains natural ingredients instead. You are far better off with the real thing—e.g., butter or olive oil—instead of margarine, real soup instead of dried soup mix, and if you must give in to the urge, homemade cookies instead of store-bought.

Know Your Fat Options

Now that you know which fats to avoid, let us discuss what your fat options are and how to best use them. Without getting too technical, fats can be either saturated or unsaturated. Whether a fat is saturated or unsaturated has to do with its mole-cular structure. Fats are composed of a series of carbon atoms strung together like cars on a train, attached by a high-energy bond. Attached to this train of carbon atoms are hydrogen atoms, along with some oxygen atoms and a carbon compound called glycerol. There are only four possible available sites on each car-bon atom where other atoms can connect. The carbon-to-carbon connections take up the first available sites, with the remaining sites filled up by the hydrogen atoms. The glycerol just attaches to the front of the train, like an engine; the oxygen attaches to the rear like a caboose. In a saturated fat the carbon molecules are connected to each other by a single bond that looks something like this: (glycerol)-C-C-C-C-C-C-(oxygen). Since only one bond connects these carbon molecules, there are still a couple of open sites on each carbon atom to which extra hydrogen atoms can attach. In a saturated fat hydrogen atoms affix themselves to these empty bonding sites on the carbon molecule, thus filling up all the available sites. Saturated fats get their name from the fact that the carbon atoms are "saturated" with these hydrogen atoms. Because they are saturated with these hydrogen atoms, they tend to be solid and firm at room temperature.

On the other hand, in an unsaturated fat, some of the carbon atom "cars" are connected to each other by a double chemical bond, which looks like this: (glycerol)-C=C-C-C=(oxygen). The double bonds between some of the carbon atoms reduce the number of potential hydrogen-bonding sites. Thus, unsaturated fats get their name from the fact that they are "not as saturated" with hydrogen atoms. There are two types of unsaturated fats. Unsaturated fats that have only one double bond between the carbon on the molecular train are called monounsaturated fats. Unsaturated fats with two or more double bonds between the carbon on the molecular train are called polyunsaturated fats. Unsaturated fats, on the other hand, because they are not saturated with hydrogen atoms, tend to liquefy at room temperature—corn oil, a liquid at room temperature, becomes a stick of margarine when hydrogenated.

Now you can picture how hydrogenation transforms polyunsaturated oil into trans-fatty margarine. It does so by chemically tearing apart the double bond between the carbon atoms in the polyunsaturated fat, thus creating additional bonding sites to which more hydrogen atoms can attach along the molecular train. Hydrogenation thus "saturates" the previously unsaturated oil with hydrogen atoms, making it a solid at room temperature.

Saturated Fats

The food sources of saturated fats include animal products such as beef, lamb, pork, and poultry; egg yolks and dairy fats such as butter, milk, cream, and cheese; and vegetable sources such as in coconut and palm oil. Vegetable shortening and margarine containing the trans-fatty "hydrogenated" oils mentioned above are also considered "saturated" in that they, too, hold as many hydrogen atoms as possible.

Saturated fats seem to have been singled out as the main culprit in heart disease, cancer, and diabetes. One of the reasons has to do with the fact that saturated fats contain aracadonic acid, which is considered an omega-6 fatty acid, otherwise known as an n-6 fatty acid. As you will see, when your consumption of foods containing omega-6 fatty acid substantially exceeds those of other omega fatty acids (n-3 and n-9), you dramatically increase the risk of degenerative diseases. Another reason saturated fats appear to be dangerous is because most foods that have saturated fats (meat, dairy products, and poultry) are potent acid-formers and can overacidify the body, putting it at risk for a vast array of chronic ailments.

While most health experts recommend you avoid excessive amounts of saturated fat in your diet, some saturated fat is necessary. The aracadonic acid contained in saturated fats gets converted to a prostaglandin (a hormonelike substance) and serves as an inflammatory agent, which is essential for natural healing and health. For example, if you slam your finger it needs to swell in order to protect it from further harm until antiinflammatory agents (a product of prostaglandins derived from unsaturated fats) can take over and continue the healing process. This inflammatory/antiinflammatory balance is part of the natural healing process.

Polyunsaturated Fats and Oils

The major food sources of polyunsaturated fats and oils are most vegetables and their oils, including safflower, sunflower, soybean, and corn oil.

Polyunsaturated oils tend to be the most unstable of all fats, meaning they are susceptible to breaking down and oxidizing.

When fats oxidize, they can produce harmful free radicals. Free radicals are unstable molecules that damage cellular structures, especially the outer fatty of the cells, proteins, membranes, and even DNA. Excessive free-radical production speeds up the aging process and causes degenerative diseases, including cancer, diabetes, liver disease, heart disease, Parkinson's disease, Alzheimer's disease, AIDS, and arthritis.

The healthiest way to get your polyunsaturated fats is in the form of fresh vegetables rather than from vegetable oils. Should you choose to use vegetable oil, follow the handling tips outlined at the back of this chapter.

While vegetable oils may also contain small amounts of the omega-6 fatty acids found in saturated fats, real vegetables are so rich in phytochemicals high in antioxidant and vitamin and mineral content that they offer powerful protection against most chronic diseases. The vegetables that seem to have the most salutary effect when it comes to chronic disease prevention are raw vegetables in general, onions, green leafy vegetables, broccoli, carrots, cabbage, brussels sprouts, and tomatoes. Garlic, parsley, ginger, soybeans, and cilantro in particular seem to possess the highest anticancer effect.

Monounsaturated Fats and Oils

The chief food sources of monounsaturated fats and oils are olive oil, flaxseed oil, peanut oil, almonds, macadamia nuts, tahini (mashed sesame seeds and olive oil), fish oils, beans, and avocados.

One negative aspect of monounsaturated oils is that they, too, are somewhat unstable but nowhere near as unstable as the polyunsaturated oils. Follow the same procedures for storing—out of direct sunlight, in a cool, dark place—as you would for other oils. You can cook with monounsaturated oil, but only on a low flame or burner. Excessive heat will oxidize the oil.

Most experts agree that of all the kinds of fat available, monounsaturated fats are by far the best for you. Most monounsaturated fats contain extraordinarily beneficial fatty acids called omega 3 or omega 9, also known as n-3 and n-9 fatty acids. The n-9 fatty acids found in olive oil, along with the n-3 fatty acids found in cold-water fish such as salmon, sardine, mackerel, halibut, cod, and tuna and present in flaxseed (linseed) oil, represent two of the most powerful guardians against the damaging effects of free radicals. Current research indicates that a diet with a high proportion of n-3 and n-9 fatty acids and a lower proportion of n-6 fatty acids provides the greatest protection against the development of a wide range of illness and diseases. Conditions as far ranging as cancer, heart disease, arthritis, chronic pain, lupus, respiratory diseases, chronic gastrointestinal diseases, diabetes, psychiatric illnesses such as schizophrenia and depression, and the common affliction of gingivitis are linked by one single thread— an imbalance of n-3 to n-6 fatty acids. Dr. David Seaman, a noted authority on health and nutrition—and someone whom I have had the pleasure of getting to know personally and whom I respect deeply—puts these findings in perspective. After researching this subject exhaustively in his fabulous textbook *Clinical Nutrition,* Seaman claims that "the great majority of chronic diseases which strike down modern man are driven, in part, by an excessive intake of n-6 fatty acids and a deficient intake of n-3 fatty acids."

Of the monounsaturated fats, olive oil and fish oils can be singled out as true champions when it comes to guarding health and well-being. Not only is olive oil rich in omega 9, it, too, is rich in phytochemicals, the highest concentration of which is found in extra-virgin olive oil. I highly recommend that you use extra-virgin olive oil in place of butter, lard, margarine, or other oils. Though research may not be considered definitive, many studies suggest that olive oil, combined with fish and vegetables, may help protect against heart disease, cancer, and diabetes. Fish oil capsules containing EPA (eicosapentaenoic acid) are probably the best source of omega 3, given that much of the fish we commonly eat, salmon in particular, is farm-raised. Questions exist regarding the concentration of EPA in farm-raised fish. If you can, purchase fish that are caught, not bred; they are more likely to contain higher concentrations of this health-promoting substance.

YOUR FAT OPTIONS

SATURATED FATS   beef, lamb, pork, poultry, egg yolks, butter, milk, cream, cheese, and coconut and palm oils

POLYUNSATURATED OILS   vegetable oils such as corn, soybean, safflower, and sunflower

MONOUNSATURATED FATS   olive oil, flaxseed oil, almonds, macadamia nuts, tahini (mashed sesame seeds and olive oil), fish oils, nut oils, beans, and avocados

---

Implications for Your Diet

In light of the all you have just read, the fat-inclusion food strategy that appears to be the most life-affirming and health-promoting emphasizes eating plenty of fresh vegetables supplemented with the cold-water fish containing n-3 fatty acids and extra-virgin olive oil. De-emphasize beef, poultry, dairy, and grains and avoid processed foods and refined sugars altogether.

What this describes is very similar to what is referred to as a traditional Mediterranean diet. Its main components are vegetables, fish, olive oil, lemons, wine, and tea. Naturally low in sugar and saturated fat and rich with foods containing omega-3 and omega-9 fatty acids, the Mediterranean diet appears to offer protection against heart disease and cancer.

THE TYPICAL AMERICAN DIET AND ITS HEALTHIER MEDITERRANEAN COUNTERPART

The American Diet	The Mediterranean Diet
high in saturated fat	low in saturated fat
high in sugar	low in sugar
high in light beer	more wine rather than beer
high in coffee	more tea than coffee
high in omega-6 fatty acids	low in omega-6 fatty acids
high in trans-fatty acids	low in trans-fatty acids
high in starchy carbohydrates and baked goods	low in starchy carbohydrates and baked goods
low in water consumption	higher in water consumption
low in extra-virgin olive oil	high in extra-virgin olive oil
extremely low in omega-3 fatty acids	high in omega-3 fatty acids
extremely low in vegetables	high in vegetables

Winning Strategies

GUIDELINES FOR CHOOSING FATS IN YOUR DIET

About one-third of your daily caloric intake can come from fats as long as the bulk of your fats come from foods that contain monounsaturated fats, monounsaturated oils, and polyunsaturated oils. The amount of monounsaturated fats and polyunsaturated fats in your diet should at least double your saturated fat consumption. This will insure a low ratio of n-6 fatty acids to n-3 and n-9 fatty acids. Most research indicates the desirable n-6 to n-3/n-9 ratio be no higher than five or four to one. Currently, the n-6 to n-3/n-9 ratio in Western civilization ranges anywhere from ten to one to twenty-to-twenty-five to one. Evidence exists that our ancestors evolved on a diet where the ratio was approximately one to one. Your objective is to keep this ratio as low as possible and eat more foods containing n-3 and n-9 fatty acids and less foods with n-6 acids. Vegetables, because of their protective qualities, are a special category and should be consumed freely and regularly. Consider them the main staple of your diet.

OMEGA-3 AND OMEGA-9 FOODS (N-3 AND N-6 FATTY ACIDS)

Eat more of these omega-3 and omega-9 rich foods or supplement with fish-oil capsules containing EPA: salmon, sardine, mackeral, halibut, cod, and tuna, extra-virgin olive oil, flaxseed (linseed) oil.

Eat less of these omega-6 rich foods: beef, lamb, pork, poultry, egg yolks, butter, milk, cream, cheese, and coconut and palm oils.

HANDLE OILS WITH CARE: SOME TIPS FROM YOUR COACH

Storing oils:

Both polyunsaturated and monounsaturated fats are somewhat unstable and can oxidize, producing the harmful free radicals we discussed earlier. Sunlight and heat can speed up the oxidation process. To protect your oils, store them out of direct sunlight and in a cool, dark place. Once opened, put them back in your refrigerator. Sometimes mixing in a few drops of vitamin E, which acts as a natural preservative and can be purchased at your local health food store, will extend the life of your oil by a few weeks. Better yet purchase oil in smaller-sized bottles, and use them within a month.

Cooking with oils:

Polyunsaturated oils are considered the least stable of all the oils and the most likely to break down and oxidize. For this reason I do not cook with polyunsaturated oils. When using a monounsaturated oil such as olive oil, cook over a moderate low flame. When cooking over a higher flame, use butter exclusively. Butter, which contains saturated fat, can withstand the additional heat, since saturated fat is the most stable of all the fats. As a general rule, I prefer grilling, broiling, or baking over pan cooking with oil.

Purchasing oils:

Always buy the highest grade cold-presser or cold-pressed oils possible. Oils that have been heated have been treated, usually with chemicals, to keep them from going rancid. The best olive oils are labeled "extra virgin." Virgin olive oil, if available, has a slightly higher acid content than does extra virgin, which may affect its taste. Olive oils marked "pure," ironically, are the lowest grade of oil. They are best left on the shelf along with those diluted oils (did anyone in the marketing department say "low fat"?) marked as "light" or "lite."

The next time you hear that a particular food has fat in it, I hope that, in light of what you've just read, your first response will be to ask, "What kind of fat is it?" instead of automatically pushing it away. Develop an awareness of the balance of fat in your diet. If you do choose to eat meat, offset your ingestion of the saturated fat and the omega-6 fatty acids it contains by supplementing your diet with fish-oil capsules. Another option is to emphasize eating foods rich in omega-3 and omega-9 fatty acids over the course of the next few days. So on Saturday, if you have a steak, focus on eating lots of fresh vegetables, salads with olive oil dressing, and maybe some fresh fish for the bulk of the next week. Emulate the

Mediterranean diet. Base your meals around vegetables, and reduce or eliminate your intake of sugar, starchy carbohydrates, and baked goods. Drink plenty of water, moderate your consumption of alcohol and coffee, choose foods rich in omega-3 fatty acids, and eliminate all trans-fatty acids. Use olive oil instead of butter. If you're dining out or traveling, request olive oil with your salads rather than rely on whatever oil may best suit the chef. Better yet, you might want to do as I do and carry a small vial of extra-virgin olive oil, just in case.

The bottom line is, there's no reason to be afraid of fats. Before you reach for something that's labeled "low fat," I'd like you to think "sugar rich" and read the next chapter.

22

Banish Sugar from Your Diet

Now that you know that fats are your friends, not your enemy, let's focus on the real adversary of the endurance athlete—sugar. Given what I've seen and experienced, I'm tempted to conclude that sugar may be single-handedly responsible for extinguishing the flame of our own innate power and stimulating the growth of modern degenerative disease. While not going quite that far, other health and fitness experts express alarm at the widespread use of sugar in modern world. The statistic heard most often is that Americans consume more than a hundred pounds of sugar a year. Just stop for a second and picture that one pound bag of sugar you see at the grocery store and imagine consuming twice that amount each week over the course of your life.

I'm not alone in my contempt about sugar. Gary Null, Ph.D., a renowned health expert, said that if sugar were invented today, the Food and Drug Administration would ban it, probably not only because of its insidious drain on our natural energy, but because of its detrimental effect on our health. Yet it is everywhere—and I'm not talking about the sugar you spoon into your iced tea, eat in your afternoon cookie, or pour in your coffee. I'm talking about sugar that lies out of our immediate sight, concealed within ketchup, tomato sauce, salad dressing, breads, crackers, juice drinks, deli meats, and cooked fruits and vegetables. When fat is removed from those muffins you eat in the morning or the yogurt you enjoy at lunch, what do you think is added to make them taste better? Why sugar, of course. And if it is not sugar that gets added, it is concentrated fruit juice or corn syrup, which gets converted to—you guessed it—sugar! Many of you may be sensitive to the issue of sugar and have tried jumping over to honey, maple syrup, and even fructose. These products still move your body in the direction of secreting insulin, burning sugar, and storing fat. Even worse is the tendency to replace fats with artificial sweeteners in an attempt to save calories (I will address this in a moment).

Runners especially have been hit hard with marketing campaigns telling them that a wide variety of sugar-based gels, bars, and drinks will give them energy during an endurance event. To some extent, the campaigns are right, and the evidence they produce to support their claims makes sense. If you depend on sugar for energy, you will be bolstered by repeated doses of it. Take the sugar away, and your performance will suffer. Probably you've personally benefited from an energy jolt after a midafternoon power bar or from a sugary gel at the twenty-mile point in a race. I have no doubt of the immediacy of the energizing effect. It's real. These energy products are potent and work, which is why people buy them—and become dependent on them.

Just because these products generate instantaneous energy and people use them doesn't mean they're good for you. Relying on sugar doesn't move you in the direction of generating energy from within. Sugar takes your power away by making you believe that you can't do it alone. It reduces the meaning of movement to a performance outcome and shrinks the expanse of experiential possibilities. No longer is the physical process about discovering who you are and gaining insight into what your body wants to be; it has become about running a faster time or getting just one more thing accomplished at the expense of realizing your long-term endurance potential. Our obsession with the outcome entraps us into a dependency on sugar and diminishes the probability that the experience of moving will uncover a new insight into how much power we actually have. By challenging yourself to step out of this dependency cycle, you put yourself in a position to free yourself from one more limiting belief.

I'm running with Frank, approaching the twenty-mile point of his first marathon. We're passing through a corridor of aid tables overflowing with packages of sugary gels, energy bars, sugary drinks, and water. We are aware of all the runners around us, frantically grabbing for one last shot of energy as they make their way along the final stages of the course. Scattered all about us are the remnants of wrappers used by the legions of runners who have preceded us, creating an eerie sense of moving through a city on the verge of abandonment. I can see that Frank, who has been working with me for more than a year and has made great strides in his sugar-free life, is tempted to partake of this mass ritual. Finally, not unexpectedly, he turns to me and asks what I think about his doing what everyone else was doing and consuming some of the gel that has just been handed to him.

"How about we don't ask me," I tell him. "We ask your body." I grab a packet of sugary gel, and we move to the side of the road to perform a muscle test. First, as we've done so many times together, Frank stands with his weight evenly distributed, lets his left arm hang comfortably by his side, and extends his right arm perpendicular to his body. I tell him to first relax and then resist as I apply gradually increasing pressure to his right arm. Both Frank and I are aware of how strong his muscle feels. Next, I ask him to hold the sugary gel in his left hand. I tell him again to relax and then resist while awaiting with detached curiosity for the message from within. He again extends his right arm, and I apply the same gradually increasing pressure to his arm—almost instantaneously his arm weakens. Frank pauses for a brief moment, looking down at the gel in his hand, looks back up at me, and smiles as he throws the gel on the ground and resumes his journey to the finish.

In one critical moment, Frank could have compromised his integrity and belief in his body by mimicking the masses and filling his body up with sugar. Instead he chose to turn away from this overwhelming temptation in order to realize an infinitely profound truth. He didn't need the sugar. He was capable of realizing his dream on his own.

From this moment on, I encourage you to recognize the pervasiveness of sugar dependency in our culture and in your own life. Your options are to eliminate sugar from your diet, dramatically reduce it, or simply take one sugary-laden item out of your life each and every day. Whatever approach you take, as long as you move in the direction of accessing the energy from inside of you, rather than from the outside, you will be successful. Or course, you can also decide to not do anything and continue on your current course. But I do want to be clear about this: eating sugar forces you to burn sugar and moves you away from the staying power of fat. It depletes your body of vital vitamins and minerals and produces acids that undermine your health. You owe it to yourself and your body to get sugar out of your life as best as you can.

Eat Sugar; Burn Sugar

Sugar—especially refined simple sugars and the high-glycemic, starchy, and concentrated carbohydrates in baked goods, most grains and grain-based foods, and certain fruits—triggers insulin production. As explained earlier, when you eat a lot of sugary foods you run the risk of entering a carbohydrate intolerant or even insulin-resistant state that provokes elevated insulin levels in the blood. A raised insulin level is the enemy of a healthy fat-burning system; it can wreck havoc on the stability of your blood sugar. Low blood sugar affects your energy, mental clarity, and ability to remain focused and alert. As insulin levels rise, all the organs of the body begin to take their energy from sugar, not fat. Your heart, liver, lungs, and muscles all are lured into a sugar-dependent state and away from the staying power of fat. Sugar—especially the refined, high-glycemic, dense and starchy carbohydrates that I am asking you to avoid—lures your body into a sugar-burning state.

Eat Sugar; Lose Vital Nutrients

Sugar not only leads your body away from its natural desire to burn fat, it depletes the body of important vitamins and minerals, including B-complex vitamins, magnesium, and chromium.[1] The B-complex vitamins serve a key role in energy metabolism, hemo-globin synthesis, and red blood cell production. Magnesium plays an important role in energy production and activating enzymes involved in protein synthesis. Magnesium deficiencies have been linked to excessive free-radical production,[2] thickening of the blood,[3] increased lactic-acid formation, and disruption of your body's ability to burn both fat and sugar.[4] A deficiency in magnesium seems to trigger a response that makes the body further deplete its magnesium stores.[5] What happens is the loss of magnesium drains the body of energy and limits muscle and tissue growth, which generates stress, which triggers more magnesium loss. Chromium is an essential trace mineral necessary for both sugar and fat metabolism. Relevant to what you now know about the dangers of insulin, chromium seems to enhance the body's sensitivity to this sugar-burning/fat-storing hormone. With chromium present, the body may be require less insulin to accomplish its task of escorting sugar into the tissue cells so that it can be burned to produce energy.

However, eating sugar can jeopardize whatever precious little chromium you have. When you lose chromium, you may hinder the ability of insulin to carry out its task and thereby induce the release of more insulin, which moves you one step closer to the carbohydrate-intolerant/insulin-resistant state. Combine these factors and you have a recipe for undermining your health and reducing your body's energy-producing potential. There is only one conclusion: for your energy's sake, stay away from sugar!

Eat Sugar; Undermine Your Health

When you eat sugar, you weaken your body's immune system, making you more vulnerable to colds and flus.[6] Robert Young, Ph.D., a research microbiologist based in Alpine, Utah and director of InnerLight Research Foundation, puts a slightly different twist on the impact sugar ingestion has on immune-system function. He claims that the health and energy challenges that arise from sugar ingestion stem from the fact that consumption of sugar is acid-forming. The acids produced from the ingestion of sugar in all its various sources, including fruits and even in the lactose in dairy products, initiates what Dr. Young calls a "cycle of imbalance." The overacidification of the blood and tissues ferments sugars, proteins, and fats rather than assimilating them or metabolizing them for energy. In this state of fermentation, the body's natural cleansing process slows down and fosters a fertile breeding ground for the development of disorganizing disease forms such as viruses, bacteria, yeast, and fungi. These disorganizing life forms then excrete their toxic waste products into the blood, causing it to become even more acidic, poisoning the surrounding tissue cells, destroying DNA, and facilitating the growth of even more disorganizing forms. Dr. Young believes that it's not that the sugar disables the immune system's ability to fight—it's just being overwhelmed and drowned by an enemy growing from within. The immune system can't keep up with the disorganizing growth going on around it. In effect, the body itself is generating the very enemy against which it is trying to defend.

This isn't such a good place to be. Overacidification leads to low energy and poor digestion, constipation, diarrhea, or inconsistent bowel movement. You may feel bloated, gain weight, or experience regular fluctuations in your weight. Overacidification can affect your mental faculties. You may suffer a lack of clarity in your thinking, have difficulty remaining focused and attentive, or encounter annoying bouts of forgetfulness, irritability, or anxiety. You might experience bodily aches, nagging pains, and discomforts that just don't seem to go away. You might become subject to more frequent illness or to the sense that you are always coming down with a cold or flulike symptoms. Telltale signs that your body is overacidified are deep dark bags under your eyes or the pale and lusterless tonality of your skin.

Overacidification of the blood can affect the strength of your bones. When you throw off the acidity/alkalinity balance of your body, you force your body to search for ways to neutralize the acids accumulating in the blood. One way your body does this is by leaching calcium from the bone. For this reason, drinking milk may not be as much of a factor in maintaining bone mineral density as it is made out to be. Your body converts the lactose in the milk into lactic acid, which acidifies the blood and siphons calcium from the bone. This is not exactly the issue that gets discussed in the dairy industry's famous "Got milk?" commercial.

Overacidification may be the reason that so many people seeking to lower their cholesterol aren't successful on a high-carbohydrate, low-fat diet. In spite of research that questions the prevailing belief that the ingestion of cholesterol, specifically from eggs, raises cholesterol levels in the blood, [6,7] most people continue to believe that high cholesterol in the blood is the result of too much cholesterol in the diet. The reality is that the 300 to 500 mg of cholesterol you might consume by eating a few eggs is miniscule compared to the

3,000 to 5,000 mg your liver can produce in response to the toxicity in your body system that can result from overacidification of the blood. The body produces cholesterol in order to protect itself from the danger of increased acid accumulation in the blood. No wonder so many people with elevated cholesterol levels find little or no relief from these conventional dietary adjustments.

Dr. Young contends that acid formation may be a major factor underlying fat retention and weight gain. Fat storage may indeed be the body's way of protecting the inner organs from the corrosive effect of the overacidification of the blood. Even the attempt to get around the sugar issue by using an artificial sweetener can lead to the same result. Nutrasweet, according to Dr. Young, gets broken down into formaldehyde, which, like the acid formed by regular table sugar, binds with fat and gets stored in your body.

The way to reverse the cycle of imbalance is to alkalize and balance the system. Our bodies were designed to operate on a diet of 70 percent alkaline foods and 30 percent acidic foods. Most people's diets are inverted. The average American eats 80 to 90 percent acidic foods and 10 percent alkaline foods.[8] If you are concerned about the levels of acidity in your blood or have experienced any of the symptoms mentioned above, I strongly urge you to find a qualified microscopist (see Appendix) who can examine your blood and help you begin the process of alkalizing and balancing your body.

Acid-Forming Foods

fruits	(all, except those listed under Alkalizing Foods)
grains	(wheat, brown rice—too much mold, and bacterial and fungal forms)
nuts	(peanuts and cashews—too much mold, and bacterial and fungal forms)
roots	(potatoes)
meat, poultry, and fish	(all, except those listed under Alkalizing Foods)
breads and baked goods	(all, except those listed under Alkalizing Foods)

dairy	(all milk and milk products, including butter or margarine)
beverages	(coffee, alcohol, soda)

Alkalizing Foods

vegetables	(especially good are cucumbers, spinach, wheat grass, endive, watercress, chives, leeks, and dandelion)
roots	(radishes, turnips, carrots, beets)
fruits	(lemons, limes, tomatoes, avocado, grapefruit, figs)
grains	(soy flour, buckwheat, millet, spelt, lentils, lima beans, fresh soy beans, basmati rice, jasmine rice)
breads and baked goods	(only live-sprouted grain products that are yeast free)
nuts	(filberts, almonds, brazil nuts)
seeds	(sunflower, sesame, flax)
oils	(flax, marine, borage, primrose, olive)
fish	(cold-water fish rich in omega 3, such as fresh salmon, mackerel, cod, trout, tuna, and halibut)
beverages	(water, green drink—either fresh vegetable juice made up of the vegetables listed above, or the Super Greens powder)

The Story of Theresa—the Acid Producer

Theresa is referred to me by her physician, who says she must start to get some exercise and begin to lose weight. She is in her late twenties, stands five feet six inches, weighs about two hundred pounds, and she has two kids. Theresa has been trying to follow a low-fat diet, but hasn't been getting anywhere. She's heard that running is good for losing weight and wants to learn how.

I ask Theresa about her lifestyle—what is her typical day like and how stable is her energy level. She gripes that she's tired all the time, which she doesn't understand because she sleeps at least eight hours a night. She barely has enough energy to get through the day, let alone enough to even think about running. She doesn't feel like running anyway: her legs are tight, her back is in pain, and her feet are swollen.

Physically, she appears tired, with pale skin and dark bags under her eyes.

Between her work and children, Theresa is home most of the time, which she enjoys; but being in close proximity to her kitchen and refrigerator has become a major distraction. She's always thinking about food. She can't go for much more than an hour without snacking. She thinks there is something wrong with her because she believes she doesn't have the willpower to stay out of the fridge. The thought that she is so lacking in discipline makes her feel worse and causes her to eat even more.

I tell her I am absolutely certain she is strong and determined; that she just hasn't discovered the right strategy yet. I address the issue of running first and suggest we don't get hung up on running just yet. For now, as long as she is moving comfortably and regularly, even if that means going out for a walk, that is fine.

We then get into the specifics of her diet, and I discover that there does seem to be a plan underlying her actions. Her doctor has expressed concern about her blood pressure, which is over the recommended upper limit of 140/90. He warns her that he will have to put her on blood-pressure medication unless she follows his advice and stops eating meat and whole-fat dairy products and adding salt to her food, which she agrees to do. She doesn't eat eggs out of concern for her cholesterol, which has now risen to a personal high of 210/40. Theresa, like many other clients when I first meet them, expresses pride at eating only products that say low or no fat on the label, including low-fat muffins, low-fat cookies, low-fat salad dressing, low-fat ice cream, diet soda, and artificial sweeteners in her coffee. She thought that the fat in her diet was making her overweight.

I say to Theresa, "I totally understand your thinking. Most people think this way. What I would like you to do is to consider the possibility that there might be another explanation for what's going on." I explain that by removing fat from her diet, she increases the probability that her body will secrete more insulin. The rise in insulin will convert into fat any sugar not immediately used for energy or fortunate enough to get stowed away in the limited storage space the body has available for sugar. To compound the dilemma, the sugary low-fat foods that comprise the bulk of her entire diet are not only causing insulin secretion, they're forming acid. Sugars, by nature, produce acid when metabolized for energy. Diets high in sugar-based products alter the natural acidity/alkalinity balance of the body, moving the body into a state of increased acidosis. I explain to her that myriad health and energy challenges arise as the body turns more acidic. These include the growth of yeast, bacteria, parasites, candida, and viruses, which can impair the immune system, drain energy, and threaten the integrity of internal organs and glands. In response, the body must then produce cholesterol and triglycerides to protect it from the corrosive effects of its acidic state. The dynamic of sugar ingestion and the insulin secretion and acid formation that follows might explain how someone on a low-fat, low-cholesterol diet feels tired all the time and experiences a rise in blood pressure and cholesterol, triglyceride, and body weight. The body is designed to protect itself from acid by binding acids to fat, which leads to fat retention and storage. No wonder Theresa's body is stuck where it is and her energy levels are getting worse.

I start by advising Theresa to immediately stop eating all nonfat, low-fat, and fat-substitute products. In their place, she is to consume as much of any green vegetable she likes, with a special emphasis on highly alkalizing (deacidifying) foods such as cucumbers, wheat grass juice, endive, celery, spinach, radishes, parsley, and kale. I tell her she can go ahead and snack on any of the foods we've just identified and not battle the desire to eat. As long as she avoids baked goods, wheat products, fruits and fruit juices, sugar, and unsprouted grains—foods that promote insulin secretion and acid formation—she can eat as much and as often as she'd like. This is a tremendous relief to her because she gets to give up the battle between herself and her urges. She now realizes that her losing battle with her appetite had nothing to do with willpower. Her eating habits had made her dependent on high-carbohydrate foods, thus her biochemistry, not her mind, was responsible for her constant need to eat.

To round off her vegetable-based meals, she chooses from the following foods: sweet potatoes, rice, quinoa (a high-protein grain), live-sprouted grains, squash, cabbage, cabbage juice, turnips, and beets. To facilitate her use of fat as an energy source, she has a teaspoon of cold-pressed flaxseed oil with each meal. She uses the fat-burning salad dressing on her salads and snacks on celery smeared with almond butter and sprouted wheat tortillas wrapped around steamed or lightly sautéed vegetables sprinkled with olive oil.

I ask Theresa to remain on this alkalizing diet for a week to 10 days. Throughout her cleansing, she continues to stay away from all starchy carbs and create each meal around vegetables. As a general rule, Theresa fills her plate up first with salad and vegetables and then adds small to moderate amounts of fish, sprouted grains, legumes, and beans. This is in direct contrast with what she used to do, which was to fill her plate up first with starchy foods and add her vegetables and salad as an afterthought. Within twelve weeks, she's lost more than twenty pounds, three inches off her waist and has gotten to the point when she can add a little running to her daily walks and still remain in a comfortable, aerobic, fat-burning state. She checks in with her physician and discovers her blood pressure, originally measured at 150/100, has now dropped to 138/85 and her cholesterol level is down to a much more respectable 190/60.

[1]J. Kron, F. A. Taylor, and E. M. Larson. *The Whole Way to Allergy Relief and Prevention* (Point Roberts, WA: Hartley and Marks, 1991).

[2]R. Elin. "Magnesium: The Fifth but Forgotten Electrolyte." *American Journal of Clinical Pathology* 102, no. 5 (1994): 616–22.

[3]M. Seelig. "Consequences of Magnesium Deficiency on Enhancement of Stress Reaction; Preventive and Theraputic Implications (a review)." *J Am Coll Nutr* 13, no. 5 (1994): 429–446

[4]Abraham G. Flechas. "Management of Fibromyalgia: Rationale for the Use of Magnesium and Malic Acid." *J Nutr Med* 3 no. 1 (1992): 49–59.

[5]Seelig 1994.

[6]M. A. Flynn, G. B. Nolph, T. C. Flynn, R. Kahrs , and G. Krause. "The Effect of Dietary Egg on Human Serum Cholesterol and Triglycerides." *American Journal of Clinical Nutrition* 32 (1979): 1051–57.

[7]H. V. Vorster, A. J. Benade, H. C. Barnard, et al. "Egg Intake Does Not Change Plasma Lipoprotein and Coagulation Profiles." *American Journal of Clinical Nutrition* 55 (1992): 400–410.

[8]R. Young. *The Bodycology System and Diet* (Innerlight International, 1998).

23

The Promise of Protein

When I was a collegiate wrestler, the customary practice was to eat steak and eggs about three hours prior to a match. We believed protein helped to make our bodies strong and sustained our will to compete. We followed this dietary practice and survived; we even thought that we thrived. Now, a red meat is the last thing in the world I would consume so close to an athletic event. During the latter stages of my multiday running career, I lived off of vegetable soup. For protein, I'd eat an egg, supplemented with a small piece of fish or water-soaked nuts or seeds. I eat pretty much the same way today, with more of an emphasis on vegetables.

In the recent past, with so much of the discussion centered on carbs for energy or the impact of dietary fat on weight gain and health, the issue of protein tended to get neglected. Today, however, protein is gaining a much higher profile as many health and fitness experts question the value of a high-carbohydrate diet, and people are more likely to fill in the void with protein rather than fat. High-protein diets are in vogue right now—whether aided by whey-based protein supplements or meals centered on meat, poultry, and eggs. However, not everyone is enamored with high-protein diets. Some are concerned about the high levels of acidity they produce, the saturated fat they deliver to the body, and whether the body needs all this protein in the first place. Vegetarians in particular contend that the body not only needs less protein but that protein from vegetables, beans, nuts, and seeds is far superior to animal sources in terms of extending youthfulness and longevity.

For me, I am happiest when my eating strategies, while revolving around fresh vegetables, include some sources of protein from fish and animal products. Whether at home or traveling, I carry a large Tupperware bowl filled with romaine lettuce, radicchio, spinach, cucumbers, broccoli, and red, green, and yellow peppers. To the full bowl of vegetables—and I do mean full—I add a small layer of protein, usually one or more of the following: grilled salmon, seared tuna, sardines, eggs, tofu, seeds, and nuts. This eating style serves me equally well for breakfast, lunch, dinner, or snacks. My energy seems the best and most consistent when I follow this pattern. Periodically, on a special occasion or during a festive event, I will enjoy a piece of red meat or fresh-roasted organic turkey.

I've resolved that a diet that includes fish and the infrequent indulgence in meat works best for me, though I'm aware that some question the healthfulness of eating any meat at all. I deal with the question of whether humans should eat in the same way that I dealt with it earlier in regard to saturated fat. My intent is not to resolve the issue here. I know vegetarians who are healthy, vibrant, and full of life, and I know meat eaters who appear the same way. I also know both vegetarians and meat eaters who are weak, frail, overweight, and lacking in vital energy. Maybe the vegetarians who are not as vibrant have just not succeeded in getting their vegan strategies down correctly yet; maybe the meat eaters have not yet struck an optimal balance in their eating habits.

My role is to support and guide you along a nutritional path that will bring you enduring energy and vibrant health—not to convince you to be a vegetarian or a meat eater. Where you end up will have to be your call, and I hope it will be based on what truly meets and matches your emotional, physical, and spiritual needs.

Protein: The Foundation of All Life

Protein is the main ingredient of all our cells as well as all the chemicals in our body that keep us functioning. Proteins contain amino acids, which are the building blocks of all cellular structures. While this essential nutrient is important for cellular growth and repair, you can put yourself at risk by having too much protein in your diet. Excessive amounts of protein in the diet can induce an abnormal metabolic state called ketosis, which is highly acidic and stressful. Also, when protein ingestion gets too high, excessive amino acids are released and our friend insulin once again is called upon to police the blood and remove these excess amino acids. It does so by storing them as fat. Part of this fat storage process can be linked to the overacidification of the blood that results from a diet high in protein. As presented earlier, to protect itself from increased levels of acid, the body tends to bind the acids to fat so that they can be removed from the blood and stored as fat.

So how much protein is enough or too much? When I first became a vegetarian in the mid 1970s, there was quite a debate regarding how much protein a person needed in order to exist. My response was always, "Don't tell me what I need to exist; tell me what I need in order to excel!"

Protein needs can be determined by your activity level, percentage of body fat, and, as you will see later, even your blood type. I've seen the recommendations for the required amount of daily protein range from as little as 10 percent to as much as 40 percent of total caloric intake. To me, these upper and lower values seem to be on the extreme side, with the value that's just right for you lying somewhere in between.

The recommended daily allowance (RDA) for protein set by the Food and Drug Administration (FDA) was last set in 1989 at .75 grams per kilogram of body weight (.34 grams per pound).[1] According to the FDA, a person weighing 150 pounds would require a minimum of 51 grams of protein per day (150 × .34 = 51). Since the metabolism of one gram of protein releases about 4 calories of energy, the average 150-pound person would be required to ingest at least 204 calories of protein per day. This amounts to approximately 6 ounces of tuna or sirloin steak, 18 ounces of lentils, or 22 ounces of tofu. Depending on whom you talk to, the amount can be higher or lower. The FDA organizes its thoughts around what figure will meet the minimal needs of the majority of the population and does not take individual differences and lifestyle into consideration.

So the debate rages as to whether the RDA for protein should be changed. Many would argue that it should go up, at least to .8 grams per kilogram of body weight (.36 grams per pound). However, a growing consensus does seem to be developing around two points. Number one, it makes sense that the amount of protein is probably more dependent on your lean muscle mass, not the total body weight, which also includes metabolically inactive fat. Body fat has no protein needs, but your muscles and tissues do, so why include fat if you're trying to figure out how much protein you need. Number two, your protein requirements probably go up as your activity level rises.

When I work with a client—or organize my own diet—I do not weigh or measure food, nor do I calculate mathematically the proportions of carbohydrates, fats, or protein my client or I will eat. I pretty much just eyeball the plate. At least three-quarters of every plate is filled with low-glycemic, alkalizing vegetables. The remaining 20 to 25 percent of the plate is filled with whatever protein and occasional grain options I choose. The dietary fat comes from the protein sources and the olive oil that I pour over my salad. Another visual guideline is the size of the palm of your hand. When consuming fish, for instance, choose a piece approximately equivalent to your palm size.

The simplest approach to protein regulation is thinking in terms of supplementing your vegetables with protein rather than supplementing your protein with vegetables. Base your eating plan on vegetables, and add to this base your fats and proteins while adjusting the amount according to what seems to work for you. Keep in mind, though, that your dietary fats will most often come from your protein sources or the oils that your add to your meals. Your objective is to develop a pattern of protein selection that includes foods high in monounsaturated fats and low in saturated fats. Exert an extra effort to include plenty of protein sources with high levels of omega-3 fatty acids, *especially* important if you continue to eat meat and dairy products.

Now that you have an idea of the role of protein in your diet, let us consider the various protein sources:

Beef products, including dairy:

Remember these products are high in saturated fat and omega-6 fatty acids. If you choose to include these protein sources in your diet, keep the amount low and sufficiently balanced with foods that contain omega-3 and -9 fatty acids.

Beef and dairy products are highly acid-forming, meaning you must be extra vigilant in including highly alkalizing foods, especially vegetables, including cucumbers, spinach, wheat grass, endive, watercress, chives, leeks, dandelion, radishes, turnips, carrots, and beets. I strongly recommend that everyone who chooses to eat meat supplement his or her diet with the Super Greens drink (see Appendix) or regularly drink an alkalizing vegetable juice made up of the green vegetables listed above. Some meat affects the acid/alkalinity balance in your body more than others do. For instance, beef, pork, and veal tend to be the most acid-forming of the meats, whereas venison, lamb, and mutton are less so. Variations in acidity/alkalinity are found in poultry and dairy as well. The chart below identifies and divides protein sources according to how they affect the acid/alkalinity balance.

HOW BEEF, POULTRY, AND DAIRY AFFECT YOUR ACID/ALKALINITY BALANCE		
	ACIDIC BUT LESS SO	ACIDIC BUT MORE SO
Red Meat	venison, lamb, and mutton	beef, pork, and veal
Poultry	duck eggs, quail eggs, chicken eggs, wild duck, goose, turkey	chicken, pheasant
Dairy	clarified butter (ghee), yogurt, goat or sheep cheese, cow milk, aged cheese, soy cheese, and goat milk	ice cream, processed cheese

Quality check:

There's no denying that food contamination, bacterial growth, and the use of hormones and antibiotics exist in the beef and poultry industry. As we enter the next century, we may find ourselves questioning the quality of *all* the food we eat, not just beef and poultry but also fish and even fruits and vegetables. The best strategy to follow is to try to remain in as much control of all aspects of your meal preparation as possible. Choose the highest-quality produce and meats, practice safe and sanitary preparation and storage practices, and don't let foods remain exposed to air for excessive or unnecessary amounts of time. When eating out, make mental notes about what goes on in the restaurants. Is there soap in the restrooms? Do people handle money and then handle food? Are the food servers wearing plastic gloves, hair nets, or caps? How would you rate the overall appearance in terms of sanitation and cleanliness?

With respect to meat and poultry purchases, buy only organic, hormone- and antibiotic-free, kosher, or free-range, if possible. If that is too difficult, it might be a clue that you are better off consuming something else. I recommend you avoid ground meat. You can't be sure of its quality or what goes into it, and because it is ground, the most of the meat is exposed to air, making it a fertile breeding ground for bacterial growth and fermentation in your intestine. So if meat is your thing, you are better off cooking—or ordering—a larger solid piece and cutting it up as you eat rather than purchasing ground or sliced meat.

Fish sources:

This is my particular favorite source of protein, though I am lucky, spending most of my life on either the East or West Coast, where fresh fish is relatively easy to purchase. As mentioned earlier, cold-water fish such as salmon, sardine, mackerel, halibut, cod, and tuna are rich in omega-3 fatty acids, a higher level of which seem to ward off the development of most kinds of degenerative disease. Fish, like meat, have different acid-producing qualities.

HOW FISH AFFECTS YOUR ACID/ALKALINITY BALANCE

LOWER ACID FORMERS	HIGHER ACID FORMERS
freshwater fish, ocean fish	shellfish, squid, mussels, lobster, crab

---

Quality check:

Even though fish may provide the best source of protein in the animal kingdom, both freshwater and saltwater fish can be contaminated. With widespread pollution of our streams, rivers, lakes, and oceans, it may become harder and harder to find fish that are free of pollutants, parasitic forms, bacterial and viral growths, toxic chemicals, and heavy metals. As a general rule, avoid all bottom feeders such as flounder, sole, catfish, and crab. If you eat these fish, do so rarely. Shellfish such as oysters, clams, mussels, and scallops can be dangerous, especially when raw, since they can contain viruses, bacteria, and concentrated levels of chemical pollutants and heavy metals. Whenever you eat fish, smell it before you eat it. Fish should have a clean smell—no hint or odor or fishiness. Eat fish close to the day you purchase it; don't keep it for more than two or three days unless you're willing to freeze it. When storing fish, rinse and repack the fish in aluminum foil and plastic wrap. Keep the fish cold, and expose it to air only when you are ready to cook it. When purchasing a whole fish at the market, check its eyes. They should be clear, not cloudy. Buy the size fish you want to use, and slice it at home rather than purchase a presliced fish. The less of the fish flesh that gets exposed to the air, the less the chance for bacterial growth.

Eggs:

Cooked properly, fresh, natural and wholesome yard eggs are highly nutritious and provide high-quality protein that can build tissue integrity. Eggs are rich in minerals, lipids, lethicin, and valuable trace minerals. Poaching is the optimal cooking method because the egg heats gradually and is ready to eat when firm.

As mentioned earlier, the cholesterol found in eggs does not seem to be the main cause of higher levels of cholesterol in the body, and eggs are increasingly being recommended as an ideal protein option for vegetarians. However, Dr. Young is adamant that eggs should not be eaten because of their extraordinarily high levels of bacteria, yeast, and fungus. This is one instance among many where you may find contradictions between authorities you trust. In the end, you have to make your own decisions about which way to go. My own belief is that for people who are very active, have low body fat, don't eat red meat or fish, or who, as you will discover later, are of a particular blood type (yes, this can be a factor), the need for protein warrants the consumption of eggs.

Quality check:

Choose organic eggs if possible, and be extra diligent in your sanitary practices when handling eggs. Eggshells can contain high levels of bacteria, so wash your hands after you touch the shell. It is preferable to cook your eggs thoroughly. When you pan-fry eggs, opt for butter over oil. If you do use oil, cook the eggs over a low flame.

Seeds, nuts, and beans:

Mixtures of organic seeds or nuts can be a wonderful protein source. They tend to be juicier and plumper when left covered within distilled or spring water overnight. Throw a handful or two on your salad, or eat as a snack.

A tasty recipe for seeds involves placing one ounce each of hulled sunflower, pumpkin, squash, and sesame seeds in an eight-ounce glass and cover with water. Stir briefly so that all the seeds have a chance to sink to the bottom of the glass. Discard any seeds that float, since they might be rancid. Place the glass in a refrigerator and leave overnight. When you are ready to eat them, drain the water and put them in a plastic bag.

Quality check:

When soaking seeds in water, do not leave the seeds in the water for more than twenty-four hours to avoid the growth of mold and fungal forms. Always rinse seeds before you soak them.

SEEDS, NUTS, AND BEANS

MORE ALKALIZING	pumpkin seeds, poppy seeds, chestnuts, lentils
LESS ALKALIZING	almonds, sesame seeds, sunflower seeds, squash seeds
LEAST ACID FORMING	pine nuts, fava beans, kidney beans, pinto beans, white beans, navy beans
MOST ACID FORMING	pistachio nuts, pecans, hazelnuts, walnuts, brazil nuts

[1]*National Research Council, Recommended Dietary Allowances* (10th ed.) Washington, D.C.: National Acadamy Press; 1989.

24

How Supplements Can Boost
Your Body's Natural Power

When people ask me about nutrition, the conversation almost invariably turns to the topic of supplements. Are supplements necessary? If so, which ones do I recommend? What are the appropriate amounts?

For much of my career I was a self-professed naturalist who didn't believe in supplements. I was committed to getting whatever nutrients I thought my body needed through real foods and nothing else. Supplements don't exist in nature. There are no multivitamin trees. Vitamin C capsules aren't growing out in the fields somewhere. I was certain that I could get all the vitamins and minerals I needed through an array of fruits, vegetables, and other natural food sources. I educated myself as to which foods contained which nutrients, and I made sure I included these foods in my diet every day.

Over the years my perspective changed. I have come to believe that supplementation is not only necessary but essential for optimal health and vitality. What changed? The earth, for starters. The soil is depleted of many natural minerals, and in some areas it is full of pesticides and chemicals that can have a negative impact on our health. The air and water contain even more pollutants. Environmental stress has to have an effect on the quality of our food.

Perhaps most alarming, you cannot be certain of the nutritional value of the foods that you eat. Earlier, in the chapter on protein, I offered you a prime example when I discussed farm-raised salmon. Certainly, raising salmon under controlled conditions seems like a wonderful way to ensure an abundant and consistent supply of this health-promoting food. However, you have to wonder whether farm-raised salmon, bred on grains, have the same nutritional properties as wild salmon that grow up feeding naturally in non-polluted waters.

For all these reasons, I am convinced that supplementation can enhance your long-term health and well-being. If, like me, you decide to take dietary supplements (and I recommend you do), you must choose between two different and distinct paths: conventional and alternative. The main distinction between what I label conventional supplementation therapy and alternative supplementation therapy has to do with the initial focus of the treatment. Read on, and I will describe each approach in detail.

The Conventional Approach

Most people think of supplementation as vitamin and mineral capsules that supply nutrients when perhaps the food chain does not. Because food sources are imperfect, my recommendation is to take a daily multiple vitamin and mineral complex to ensure that you get all the nutrients you need. The second strategy that comes to mind involves nutrients that address the issue of free-radical production and oxidation of the cells. As outlined earlier, antioxidant therapies counter the effects of oxidation caused by excessive free-radical production when the body undergoes stress. Oxidation is the primary mechanism of organic degradation, especially when you exercise rigorously. When you work out at high intensities, you ventilate tremendous amounts of oxygen in and out of your body—as much as twelve to twenty times the amount that moves through the body at rest. All this oxygen can produce masses of free radicals (fragmented oxygen molecules) that create oxidative stress on healthy cell membranes. Antioxidant supplements can combat this stress on the cells. The classic antioxidants are vitamins A, C, and E. The nutrition community has also shown interest in beta-carotene (a form of vitamin A), chromium piccolinate, coenzyme Q10, melatonin, zinc, and selenium.

Two additional conventional supplementation strategies include taking nutrients to boost the body's metabolism and endurance capability, and ingesting nutrients that increase your ability to build muscle mass.

To me, conventional supplementation therapy is modeled after the conventional approach to medicine: alleviate symptoms instead of address the causes of the symptoms. Just throwing vitamins and minerals into a body that is overacidic, out of balance, and in dire need of antioxidants because of poor diet and exercise habits never addresses the cause of the symptoms, nor does it ensure that the body will be able to process and absorb the supplements in the first place.

The Alternative Approach

While conventional supplementation strategies can be effective, they overlook the degree to which a person may be either receptive or resistant to vitamin and mineral therapies. Your system's acidity/alkalinity balance determines how effective a particular supplementation strategy will be. According to Dr. Robert Young (introduced in the chapter on sugar), who is a key figure in a movement centered around what can be called "the new biology," the first step in any supplementation program is to first de-acidify, cleanse, and balance the system. Once the body is alkalized and in balance, then—and only then—can the infusion of vitamins and minerals provide the most impact. Without an optimal acidity/alkalinity balance present, much of whatever vitamin or mineral supplements get ingested will not be absorbed and their protective or life-affirming value will get lost.

According to Young, a stressful biochemical environment is caused by any disturbance that creates acids. These disturbances can be nutritional (poor eating habits); an inability to cope with and manage stress; negative thoughts, pessimism, and resignation; and either exercising too excessively (too much anaerobic sugar-burning, not enough aerobic fat-burning) or not exercising at all. By consuming alkalizing foods (mainly vegetables), moving aerobically as often as you can, and focusing on the positive aspects of your life, you can move your body toward a more alkaline and less acidic state.

Young and other proponents of a new biology contend that too much acid in the body robs the blood of oxygen. As your body loses oxygen, your metabolism slows down. This depletion of oxygen causes you to digest foods more slowly. Overacidification increases the possibility of weight gain, sluggishness, and fermentation, which creates yeast and fungi. The waste products of these organisms, called mycotoxins, can be damaging to your cells. The first focus of any supplementation strategy, according to this new biology, is to neutralize the acid in the blood. After deacidifying the body, you must cleanse it to rid the body of excess acids and wastes. The next step is to neutralize any existing mycotoxin-producing organisms. Finally, a construction phase infuses the vital nutrients to nourish the cells and repair any damage that has already occurred. After you undergo this three-step process, your body will be much more receptive to receiving, absorbing, and processing supplemental vitamins and nutrients.

Many products can deacidify, cleanse, and supply vital nutrients to your body. Ask your local health food store to recommend specific products, particularly ones that are natural and vegetable-based. In my opinion, the best product on the market is Young's

Super Greens mix, which contains natural sprouted nutrients, fibers, enzymes, amino acids, and essential minerals designed to cleanse tissues, control toxic intruders, and construct healthier cells. I urge you adopt an alkalizing lifestyle and supplement it with the Super Greens or a comparable product. If you have questions or want more information on InnerLight products, refer to the Endurance Essentials section in the back of the book.

Supplemental Strategies that Enhance Metabolism and Promote Endurance

As mentioned earlier, certain nutrients can enhance the body's ability to produce energy and burn fat. Supplements that impact energy metabolism are called lipotrophic factors and include L-carnitine, choline, chromium, and essential fatty-acid complexes. These supplements, along with beet leaf extract, can help utilize and mobilize fats and maintain a balance of total to good (HDL) cholesterol.

For all supplements, the recommended dosages vary from the FDA daily allowance to mega doses favored by some health practitioners. To determine the appropriate amounts for you, I suggest you follow manufacturer's recommended dosages or consult with your healthcare provider. Many of the supplements listed below are found in high-quality multivitamin capsules. Check the label to be sure.

L-CARNITINE

L-carnitine moves fat from the adipose (fat-storage cells) to the mitochondria (fat-burning ovens). The higher the level of L-carnitine in your muscles, the more body fat you transport to your muscles to use for fuel. Ideally, the human body makes sufficient amounts of L-carnitine; however, if you are overweight and are on a restrictive diet, your body may not produce enough

L-carnitine. Supplementation can help. When shopping for L-carnitine, purchase a reputable brand. Inexpensive or low-quality L-carnitine supplements contain racemic or dL-carnitine, which can actually interfere with L-carnitine metabolism.

Natural sources of L-carnitine: primarily red meat (lamb and beef in particular), with negligible amounts found in dairy products, vegetables, fruits, and certain cereals. Consider L-carnitine supplementation or make sure your multivitamin contains it if you choose not to eat animal products.

CHOLINE

Choline is a member of the B-complex family and a lipotrophic agent (fat emulsifier). It works with other B-complex members (specifically inositol) to utilize fats and cholesterol. Choline seems to emulsify cholesterol so that it doesn't settle on artery walls or in the gall bladder.

Natural sources of choline: soy beans, wheat germ, fish, and leafy green vegetables.

CHROMIUM

Chromium can affect the body's ability to burn fat by increasing its sensitivity to insulin. Insulin enables the body to deal with sugar, carrying it into the cells to be metabolized for energy. Insulin also plays a role in promoting fat storage. As insulin sensitivity is reduced (a condition called insulin resistance), the body must secrete more and more insulin to metabolize sugar. As insulin levels rise, so does the body's tendency to store fat, not burn it! Chromium can help counteract this process.

Natural sources of chromium: whole grains, wheat germ, and nuts.

MARINE LIPIDS, FISH OILS, AND BORAGE OIL

These oils, along with Vitamin E, contain essential omega-3 fatty acids, EPA, and DHA, which improve energy, nervous system and brain function; promote healthy skin, muscle growth, and fat usage (rather than storage), and decrease the likelihood of cardiovascular related disease. Omega-3 fats found in fish and made by your body from the alphalinoleic acid found in flax oil increases insulin sensitivity and improves fat metabolism. Most people on modern diets are deficient in omega-3 fats.

Natural sources of good oils/lipids: organic cold-pressed flaxseed oil, Dr. Udos perfected oil blend, and cold-water fish such as salmon, mackerel, trout, and sardines.

COENZYME Q10 (CoQ10)

Also known as ubiquinone, coenzyme Q10 is found in the mitochondria (fat-burning ovens) of all cells. CoQlO seems to enhance the function of the heart tissue or myocardium, building a stronger, healthier heart, which will hopefully translate into greater longevity. As you build up your cardiac strength through exercise, CoQ10 can support the function of your heart.

Natural sources of coenzyme Q10: whole grains; cold-water fish as salmon, mackerel, trout, and sardines.

MAGNESIUM

Found in whole grains and green leafy vegetables, magnesium activates enzymes involved in protein synthesis. It plays a vital role in glucose metabolism by facilitating the formation of muscle and liver glycogen from glucose carried in the blood. Magnesium is also a crucial ingredient in the breakdown of glucose, fatty acids, and amino acids. It is an important factor in the synthesis of fats and proteins and in nervous system function and muscle contraction.

Natural sources of magnesium: whole seeds, nuts, legumes and soy beans, green vegetables, including spinach and beet greens, and unmilled grains.

B Vitamins

The twenty-two known vitamins in the B-complex group work better as a group than individually. I recommend that you take a complete B-complex supplement rather than taking one or two of the twenty two.

Natural sources of B vitamins: grains, legumes, nuts, vegetables, meats, and fortified soy milk and soy products.

Glucosamine Sulfate and Chondroitin Sulfate

Glucosamine sulfate and chondroitin sulfate are involved in maintaining the elasticity and integrity of many body parts and tissues, including connective tissue, arterial walls, nails, skin, bones, ligaments, and heart valves. The only significant food source of chondroitin sulfate is animal cartilage. Glucosamine sulfate does not appear in most of the food we eat. For these reasons, I recommend supplementation, especially if you choose not to eat animal products and are engaged in regular physical training.

A Word About Creatine

Creatine, one of the most talked about supplements in the fitness world, is a muscle-building supplement that is found in the body. Approximately 95 percent of your creatine supply is in the skeletal muscles. The remaining 5 percent is spread throughout the rest of the body, including the heart and brain. Your body's ability to generate energy for muscle contractions is dependent on its supply of creatine. Creatine itself is synthesized in the liver, pancreas, and kidneys, as well as absorbed into the system through the consumption of certain foods. Foods rich in creatine include meats such as beef and pork, and fish such as tuna, cod, salmon, and herring. Creatine supplementation has become popular among vegetarians and health conscious, fitness-minded individuals who want to increase their muscle density while avoiding high-fat animal sources.

I used creatine for about a year and found it effective in inducing an increase in the size and bulk of my muscles. For me, creatine supplementation definitely had an effect. Yet I know others who did not experience any increase in the size of their muscles with creatine. (Other supplements used to increase muscle mass are whey-based products. Whey, a derivative of dairy, is not something I recommend, as you will discover in the next chapter, for those with blood type O and A.)

I believe that there are many unanswered questions about creatine—and some reason for concern. The long-term effects of creatine supplementation—especially in the high dosages taken by many bodybuilders—are still not known. Anecdotal evidence exists, not only for the benefits of creatine ingestion, but for the side effects as well. Creatine has been linked with kidney damage, cramping, muscle pulls, nausea, and diarrhea. I stopped taking creatine because I am convinced that a balanced and healthy non-acidic body can extract sufficient amounts of creatine from natural creatine sources. My philosophy is in part based on the fact that I do consume fish and sometimes meat. When I coach clients, I leave the question of creatine supplementation up to them. For vegetarians who want to bulk up the body, creatine may be an option. I have made a decision for me; you will have to make your own. In the end, I would rather focus on relying on my body's own natural resources when it comes to generating power and strength.

25

Personalize Your Food Strategies

Our exploration of nutritional strategies began with an awareness of the importance of burning fat and including fat in your diet to unlock the energy from within. We went from there to a clearer understanding of why sugar products set into motion a series of events that move you away from vitality and optimal health. The next stop on our trek brought us to protein and the critical role it plays in growth and development. Now, as our journey together draws to a close and you are about to embark on your own, it's time to draw upon the powerful distinctions made thus far and use them in a way that brings you one step closer to having enduring energy.

As you move from appreciating time-honored wisdoms of how the human body works to the more pressing realities of your day-to-day life, you might come to realize, as I have, that what works for someone else may not work for you. While coaching thousands of clients, I've seen this happen so often—two people on the same diet get different results. I've seen people thrive as vegetarians while others seem to lose vitality when they eliminate meat from their diets. There are those who cannot tolerate dairy at all, while others are perfectly fine with moderate amounts of it in their diet.

For me, these individual differences are one of the most exciting aspects of coaching. Much of the work I do with my clients revolves around using the guiding principles established in the earlier chapters as a launching point for figuring out which particular foods work best for them. We start off by getting sugar out of the diet along with most dense starchy carbohydrates, minimizing alcohol consumption, and reducing or eliminating coffee and other sources of caffeine such as black tea, cola, and chocolate. We follow that up by bringing in lots of alkalizing vegetables and drinking plenty of water. We then use the technologies such as muscle testing to determine which foods energize and which foods seem to take energy away. We monitor the hip-to-waist ratio to determine if we're moving away from a dependency on carbohydrates. We avail ourselves of technologies such as the carbon-dioxide/oxygen analyzer to monitor changes in the body's energy-producing system to see if more and more energy derives from fat, and microscopy to assess the health and function of the blood. Tracking the productivity the client displays while exercising in the most efficient pace (MEP) cardio c-quence is another excellent way to evaluate the degree to which nutritional, training, and mindset strategies enhance progress. The more energized you become, the more productive you can be while continuing to move in a state that remains attractive and comfortable to you. The end effect can be a dramatic increase in energy level, personal productivity, and general optimism and excitement about life.

As you zoom in on which specific foods to include in your diet, personal preferences come into play. Certain foods are absolutely out of the question for some people: there are those, who won't eat a particular type of fish (or any fish at all) or certain kinds of vegetables, while others can't imagine not starting the day with a bowl of oatmeal and some raisins. Back in the early 1990s, the press made a big deal out of President George Bush's abhorrence of broccoli. While your likes and dislikes might not make the national media, I'm sure your family and friends know there are certain foods that they should not serve to you. These kinds of personal signals can be most revealing, especially if you get to the point where you can be fairly confident that your attraction or aversion to a particular food is not driven by carbohydrate cravings emanating out of a sugar dependency.

There are many reasons for food preferences. You may have noticed that every time you eat a cabbage or brussels sprouts, for instance, your digestion feels a little off and your stomach gets irritated, while your friend can eat the exact same meal and feel just fine. I used to get dizzy almost every time I ate an orange, which you won't catch me doing anymore. My wife does not do well on eggplants. With other people it is meat. The stories I hear about the problems some people experience after eating meat! As I mentioned earlier on in the book, my mom doesn't seem to benefit from eating meat, though she still continues to do so, however infrequently. Like clockwork she'll eat a steak and have a restless sleep later on that night. Yet my sister and I can eat meat, sleep like babies, and wake up refreshed the following day.

The naturopath James D'Adamo first presented a theory over twenty years ago that has been particularly attractive to me, and recently I've incorporated it into my practice. During his studies of the nutritional programs offered at several prestigious European spas, D'Adamo noticed that even under these very standardized conditions, certain clients had better outcomes, both in the way they felt and the way their bodies changed. D'Adamo believed that since the body is nourished through the blood, the blood was the intervening factor, since the food was the same. From that point on in his own practice, he began typing his clients' blood to see if he could find a pattern between certain foods and patterns of blood types. Through this research he found that his patients who were type O thrived on a high-protein diet that included meat, while the type-A clients were quite the opposite, doing better on a vegetarian diet. He also noticed behavioral differences among the blood types. The Os seemed to gravitate toward more vigorous activities such as running and aerobics, whereas the As enjoyed more calming types of movement, including yoga and tai chi.

Intrigued by the findings, D'Adamo's son Peter, while finishing his studies at naturopathy school, started scanning journals in search of a connection between blood type and disease. His first breakthrough came when he found certain diseases were linked to specific blood types. Because of higher levels of stomach acid, individuals with type O blood had a greater predisposition to peptic ulcers. Individuals with type-A blood, because of lower levels of stomach acid, had a tendency to pernicious anemia (which requires higher levels of stomach acid to process) and stomach cancer. This clarified what his father had discovered: the higher acid content of the digestive system of the Os was better suited for breaking down a diet that included meat, whereas the less acidic, more sensitive digestive system of the As did better with a meat-free diet.

These observations led to an elaborate system of organizing food choice based on blood type. Peter D'Adamo has taken the mantle and furthered his father's work in his remarkable treatise, *Eat Right 4 Your Type*. In the book D'Adamo delivers a powerful message that knowing your blood type can provide a genetic blueprint to guide you to the choice of food. What unfolds is a wonderfully attractive story about how blood evolved sequentially and in relation to the food that was available during each historical epoch.

Here, according to D'Adamo, is how it works. There are four distinct blood types: O, A, B, or AB. (No special consideration are given to subdivisions—positive or negative Rh factors—of blood type.) D'Adamo drew on research that had established that all human beings started out as type Os. In fact, it is theorized that type O blood existed as far back as 500,000 B.C., fueling the system of the Neanderthal. Type O remained alone right through the time Cro-Magnon appeared around 50,000 B.C. The Cro-

Magnon were fierce and accomplished hunters who perfected weaponry and moved to the top of the food chain. They lived primarily on a diet of meat, plants, fruit, roots, and berries. They became so proficient at hunting game that they wiped out their primary food supply, forcing a migration out of northeastern Africa, the cradle of civilization that spawned them.

By 30,000 B.C., humans had wandered out of Africa and into Europe and Asia, and by 10,000 B.C. inhabited all continents save Antarctica. Somewhere around 25,000 B.C., in response to the scarcity of meat, humans began to cultivate agriculture and livestock. Instead of the nomadic search for game, humans began a more stable existence of preparing the soil and reaping the harvest of the earth, working together in communities. Now, rather than a regular diet of whatever animals they could kill or vegetation they could find, meals revolved around grains and produce that could be grown from the land. This change in lifestyle and diet seemed to favor individuals with more sensitive digestive tracts, which were better suited for a diet with more vegetables and less meat. Out of this dynamic between changes in the diet and the pattern of day-to-day life emerged what we now know as blood type A.

Human migrations continued. Around 15,000 B.C., a new blood type emerged, type B, as nomads pushed into the colder, more mountainous regions now known as Pakistan, Russia, and Mongolia. Domestication of animals brought dairy into the human food chain. According to D'Adamo, only individuals with type B blood seem to benefit from the regular consumption of dairy.

The mingling of type A and type B blood between 12,000 to 10,000 B.C. gave rise to a new and modern AB blood type. AB is rarely found in excavated gravesites prior to A.D. 900. It exists in less than 5 percent of population.

Each of the four blood types provides a distinct and permanent biochemical marker called an antigen. The antigen markers differentiate the blood types from one another; thus type O blood has a different biochemical fingerprint than type A, B, or AB blood. If you infuse the blood of a type A individual into that of a blood type O, the O blood will immediately recognize that the blood just introduced is not similar and will trigger a response that prevents the foreign blood from being accepted. The process of rejection is called agglutination, which literally means gluing. What this means is that the body recognizes that the new blood cells are "not one of us" and orders the immune system to attack the invading blood cells. The immune system does this by producing antibodies that surround and immobilize these new and differently marked blood cells by adhering to their surface and holding the invaders hostage until it they can be disposed of.

Like the blood, food carries its own antigen-like markers called lectins, which are abundant and diverse proteins. D'Adamo asserts that foods can carry lectins that are toxic, neutral, or beneficial to a specific blood type. Foods with toxic lectins promote agglutination; foods with neutral lectins deliver nutrients but do not affect the agglutination process; foods with beneficial lectins reverse the process of agglutination. Lectins have similar agglutinating properties as the blood antigens and the body jumps into action when it notices the arrival of a food carrying an incompatible lectin marker. The same process that applied to the introduction of a different blood type also applies to the food lectins. When a food containing lectins incompatible with the blood type is introduced, it, like other foods containing compatible lectins, is broken down by your digestive system. The lectins themselves, however, remain intact and settle somewhere in the body, with different lectins targeting different places of the body in which to settle. Lectins not congruent with your blood type are then identified as intruders, triggering an agglutinating response similar to what happens when blood of a different type is introduced in the body. Recognizing that the lectin is "not one of us," the body orders an attack, causing a clustering of cells around the foreign lectin marking it for destruction. For example, milk has type B properties. When a type O consumes milk, the O's body will recognize the milk as "not one of us" and immediately trigger an agglutinating response.

Incorporating the theory of blood evolution into a dietary program, D'Adamo came up with the following tendencies:

Type O:

The hunter; meat-eater; powerful digestive tract; the universal donor. Os thrive on a higher protein diet composed of meat, fish, and vegetables. Os do better on a diet that has only a moderate amount of beans and neutral grains. Os should avoid dairy and most conventional grains such as wheat and corn. Most North Americans, about 62 percent, are blood type O.

Type A:

The cultivator; the vegetarian; sensitive digestive tract. People with blood type A should base their diets on vegetables, grains, beans, legumes, soy products, fruit, and seafood; they are not good at processing dairy, meat, and most forms of wheat. Blood type A makes up about 25 percent of the North American population.

Type B:

The nomad; versatile and adaptive; balanced omnivore. People of this type benefit from a balanced diet of meat, dairy, grains, beans, legumes, vegetables, and fruits. Chicken and tomatoes are particularly toxic to type B eaters. They should also avoid corn, lentils, sesame seeds, peanut butter, peanuts, buckwheat, and wheat. About 9 percent of the North American population are blood type B.

Type AB:

The modern; designed for modern conditions. The universal recipient. The new kids on the block, AB types are a blend of A and B tendencies. They do best on a mixed diet and benefit by eating foods from all food categories. Blood type AB is the rarest of all the blood types, accounting for about 4 percent of the North American population.

What initially drew me to D'Adamo's perspective is its attempt to answer the question, "How could a diet that works so well on one person not work at all for another?" He answers by making the case that blood type might be the underlying variable. His theory, based on the evolutionary sequence to the blood, satisfies my need for a historical context. Once you acknowledge that the blood evolved in a chronological order, it's not too far of a leap to infer that an affinity might exist between the individual blood types and the kinds of foods that were available at the time they appeared.

Other aspects of the theory move me as well. I know medical doctors already follow certain rules when it comes to blood type. You can't indiscriminately transfuse blood from one person into another. You have to match them up first. You can only exchange blood between the same types, with two exceptions: Os are the universal donors, since all blood derived from Os; ABs are the universal recipients because they are the result of the intermingling of As and Bs. Is it so far removed from this medical fact to conceive that different blood types could react differently to certain foods?

In the Far East, knowing your blood type is as ordinary as knowing your birthday. It's so ingrained in the cultural consciousness that blood-type distinctions are used to recruit people for jobs. Matching blood types to job requirement is based on the observation that different blood types exhibit different personality traits. D'Adamo has found that the Os tend to be strong, self-reliant, and daring; As are cooperative, orderly, and self-restrained; Bs are flexible, creative, and balanced; and ABs are also creative, as well as sensitive and enigmatic. In my own practice, I began to see a congruency between these personality types and blood types. This becomes especially obvious when I see the relationship between a client's blood type and the type of exercise he or she likes to do—strenuous, moderate, or easy and relaxed.

The D'Adamos explain the exercise preferences in terms of the way each blood type tends to handle stress. For Os, stress goes right into the muscles, so they gravitate toward rigorous physical activity for relief. Type Os seem to require the most physical activity of all the blood types. (And if you haven't guessed, I am an O.) Type As are the opposite. They store stress in the nervous and immune systems more than the muscles and bones. For type-A people, stress can lead to anxiety and irritability, making calming activities such as golf, yoga, and Tai chi the most beneficial. Type Bs need a balance between the intense physical activity of Os and the more calming activity of As. Type ABs are more like the As and do best with calming activity. Heavy competitive sports and exercise is theorized to add to, not release, stress for ABs.

Finally, there's the issue of the food lists contained in D'Adamo's book, which are extraordinarily appealing in both their simplicity and comprehensiveness. Every vegetable, meat, grain, bean, fish, and fruit—even spices and condiments—are classified in terms of whether they are beneficial, neutral, or toxic for each blood type. In the fruit group, for instance, bananas are toxic to As, neutral to Os and ABs, and beneficial to Bs.

While the structure of D'Adamo's food lists are attractive to me, I was curious as to how he can collate such an extensive index of specific foods and the response they elicit for each blood type. The inference is that D'Adamo based his research on monitoring the reaction of blood to the systematic and controlled exposure to each and every possible food substance.

It is one thing to be intellectually fascinated with the perspective and another to have confidence in it and actually use it with clients as an additional lens through which to filter food choices. My day-to-day diet is already very akin to what D'Adamo recommends for a type O. I've already removed dairy, wheat, and most grains from my diet, which are classic O toxins. My diet, as you already know, is predominantly salad and fish. So I went ahead and tried it on myself, not expecting dramatic results. All that I needed to do is remove some of the alkalizing vegetables that I had been eating, a lot of which are considered toxic to my blood type. These included cauliflower, eggplant, avocado, brussels sprouts, alfalfa sprouts, mustard greens, and cabbage. Within a few days, I noticed subtle yet appealing changes; in particular, I was more regular in my bowel movements. The slight gastrointestinal distress I would experience when I ran disappeared when I eliminated these toxic foods. I was starting to get hooked on the blood type theory.

You probably have some idea as to where I'm going next. Filled with both the excitement of intellectual discovery and the fact that I was appreciably more comfortable when I ran—and hardly passing any gas at all, by the way—I had one additional step to take! I interrogated my body by using muscle testing to assess the validity of D'Adamo's claims. I purchased a basketful of foods based on D'Adamo's list, foods that are supposed to be toxic to some blood types and neutral or beneficial to others. My basket includes oranges, which are toxic to all blood types but B; avocados, which are toxic to all blood types but A; and potatoes, considered toxic to As and Os and neutral to Bs and ABs.

I began my experiment by having my first subject let me muscle-test her without holding anything. I identified the right shoulder muscle as a strong indicator muscle. After establishing that the muscle was strong, I handed her an orange, and I retested the muscle. It was noticeably weaker. I asked her her blood type, and she said A. I repeated the same test on her using other foods. A pattern began to develop. Foods that were toxic to As weakened her, and foods that were neutral or beneficial had little effect. I repeated this form of testing with an assortment of friends, clients, and family members. I discovered that if a person holds a food that is toxic to his or her blood type, about 85 percent of the time the arm weakens. In a sense, I'm following a similar process to D'Adamo's; but whereas he examined the response of the blood to the food lectins under a microscope, I used the muscle-testing techniques that have served me so well over the course of my career. Armed with the confidence that the muscle testing seems to verify D'Adamo's claims, I took my act on stage and made it one of the more entertaining features of my seminars. Imagine a roomful of people and up on stage are four people, one from each blood type. I go around from person to person, having him or her hold a fruit or vegetable, eliciting a wide variety of responses to the delight of the seminar participants. Sometimes I am able to get a strong, muscular type-O man up on stage and contrast him with a petite woman who is a type A. After handing the avocado to the man (toxic to an O), I test his muscle and it immediately weakens. I repeat the same exact procedure with the woman and, to the amazement of the O, her arm is strong. No surprise there—avocados are neutral to As. You can try this at home for yourself. The body is truly remarkable!

Now, to my battle cry of "eat lots of vegetables, drink plenty of water, and avoid sugar at all costs," I've added "eat according to your blood type." Blood-type distinctions are part of the core of my eating for the distance program. Most often, when I test clients and show them food lists, they respond, "Oh my gosh. Now I know why I've always liked these foods and disliked those." That comment is followed by remarks such as, "You're telling me I can't eat 'chicken' or 'meat' or 'dairy.' That's all I eat!" Finally, after looking down the blood type food lists, they begin to feel better as they spot things that they thought they shouldn't eat, and the list tells them they can.

Basing nutritional strategies on blood type allows them to further personalize their choice of foods. Karl is example of a client for whom the blood type distinction has been incredibly helpful.

For most of his adult life, Karl based his food choices on whatever he felt like eating. As a real-estate developer and karate master, he is physically and mentally strong enough to get by on a diet that is mediocre at best. His favorite meal is a big steak, a potato, and a glass of Merlot. After a long day of work, he rewards himself with a bowl of ice cream as he relaxes in front of the tube. He often works twelve-hour days fueled on mostly carbs. His only complaint is that he has irregular bowel movements.

A devotee of self-improvement, Karl keeps reading about the benefits of a healthy vegetarian diet and decides to try it out. As he approaches fifty, he's aware that the habits that sustained him for the early part of his life may not be the ones to bring him into the new millennium.

Now, as a vegetarian, Karl bases his meals around vegetables. In between meals, he snacks on fruit. He loves all the new foods in his diet and for the first time in his life he has a bowel movement every day.

In our initial session, Karl told me about his transformation, and I introduced him to the blood type distinctions. He was interested in their historical context and says that he's never understood how we all were supposed to eat the same thing. Even though he's benefiting from his current diet, he wants to try to eat according to his blood type. After our session, Karl gets his blood tested and discovers he is type B. A man who never does anything less than 100 percent, Karl eats only those foods that are either beneficial or neutral to Bs. This means giving up certain fruits, corn, avocados, and tomatoes and reintroducing meat back into his diet. He has a fresh piece of fish almost four times a week, which he loves.

For Karl, the shift from a vegetarian to a B diet takes him another step along the road to optimal health. He reports that he is able to maintain his feelings of well-being for longer and longer periods of time. He laughs more and his mind is brighter.

Perhaps most importantly, he is one step closer to understanding what works best for his body. He can eat a food and soon after know whether it arms him with or depletes him of energy. His attitude about his imminent fiftieth birthday has shifted from one of dread to "bring it on."

MEAL PLANNING FOR ALL BLOOD TYPES

Refer to the following food list when preparing meals for yourself and others.

FOOD BENEFICIAL TO ALL

Seafood	mackerel, salmon, sardine
Oil	olive oil
Breads	essene bread, Ezekiel bread
Vegetables	beet leaves, broccoli, collard greens, kale, parsley, parsnips
Fruit	plums
Herbal teas	ginger tea, rosehip tea

FOOD NEUTRAL TO ALL (OR BENEFICIAL TO SOME)

Meats and Poultry	turkey
Seafood	albacore (tuna), grouper, mahi mahi, pickerel, rainbow trout, red snapper, sea trout, sturgeon, swordfish, whitefish
Dairy and Eggs	farmer cheese, feta, goat cheese, mozzarella, soy cheese, soy milk
Nuts and Seeds	almond butter, almonds, chestnuts, hickory, macadamia, pecans, walnuts
Oil	cod liver oil, linseed (flax) oil
Beans	green beans, green peas, jicama beans, northern beans, pea pods, red soy beans, snap peas, white beans
Cereals	cream of rice, millet, rice (puffed), rice bran, spelt
Breads, Grains, and Pasta	brown rice bread, fin crisp, gluten-free bread, ideal flat bread, millet, quinoa, soy bread and flour, spelt bread and flour, spelt pasta, wasa bread, rice, basmati and white, rice cakes, rice flour, rice noodles
Vegetables	arugula, asparagus, bamboo shoots, beets, bok choy, carrots, celery, cucumber, daikon, dandelion, endive, escarole, fennel, leeks, lettuce (bibb, iceberg, romaine), mesclun, mushroom (oyster cap, portobello), okra, onions (red, Spanish, yellow),

	radicchio, scallion, seaweed, shallots, snow peas, spinach, squash (all types), swiss chard, turnips, water chestnuts, watercress, zucchini
Fruits	apples, apricots, blueberries, boysenberries, cherries, cranberries, currants (black and red), dates and figs (dried and fresh), grapes (all kinds), guava, kiwi, kumquat, lemons, melon (crenshaw), nectarines, peaches, pears, raisins, raspberries, watermelon
Spices and Condiments	apple butter, basil, chocolate, curry, dill, garlic, ginger, horseradish, mint, miso, mustard, paprika, parsley, rosemary, salt, soy sauce, tamari, tarragon, thyme
Beverages	green tea, wine (white and red)

FOOD TOXIC TO ALL

Meats and Poultry	bacon, goose, ham, pork, quail
Seafood	barracuda, conch, lox (smoked salmon), octopus
Dairy	American cheese, bleu cheese, ice cream
Oil	corn oil, cottonseed oil, safflower oil
Vegetables	black olives
Spices and Condiments	black ground pepper, white pepper, ketchup
Herbal Teas	corn silk tea, red clover tea, rhubarb tea
Beverages	distilled liquor, cola and soda (including diet soda)

As with almost any approach to nutrition, D'Adamo's theories and practices have been both lauded and denounced. Even if one were to accept many of his premises—which I do—that does not mean that you then indiscriminately follow every one of the food recommendations made for your particular blood type. Take the type O diet, for instance. Although D'Adamo maintains that Os do better with some meat in the diet, this does not mean that each and every meal you consume must have meat in it. There is ample evidence that suggests that even for the Stone Age Os, the diet consisted mainly of whatever plants, roots, berries, even grubs and insects could be found. Meat from the hunt was not a daily staple—certainly the early Os didn't dine on saber-toothed tiger for breakfast, giant sloth for lunch, and a mastodon for dinner. Meals were probably much more balanced than that. While the men were out hunting, the women were out foraging. My guess is they both ate a lot more of what the women found than what the men were able to catch. And when the men were successful at bringing home the meat, the feast was probably much different than you might expect. Certainly not like a Sunday afternoon barbecue out on the ranch. The meat was most likely eaten raw, and the organs and the brains—the highest-quality protein—were probably eaten first.

Chances are that even if you totally bought into D'Adamo's Os-as-meat-eater's strategy, you would not want to replicate the dining habits of our Stone Age type-A ancestors. Eating raw meat can be dangerous. You really must be careful of its quality and cleanliness, especially organ meats like the liver and kidneys, which filter out toxins from the body. In an age where food contamination in the meat and poultry industry is so prevalent, eating these foods can be risky if the utmost of care is not practiced.

The bottom line is that while D'Adamo's approach to nutrition may be appealing, it still does not offer a foolproof formula. You still must evaluate your options, make informed decisions, and understand that lifestyle, genetics, and conviction all play a part in determining what food choices will be most beneficial to your body.

It's a blessing in disguise that no formula or technology is foolproof. It would lead us into a false confidence that we don't have to think about or participate in the decisions that affect our lives. The significance in our lives is not found in dutifully following a formula but in our ability to go beyond formulas to discover the power that already lies within us. Rise to the challenge of constant and never-ending vigilance with your body and your life. Once you do, you will leave behind the boundaries built by the expectations of others and move to a place where there are no boundaries and you create the possibilities that are all your own.

Welcome. You've arrived. Anything—and everything—is now possible.

Stu Mittleman Recommends . . . the Endurance Essentials

Must Reads

As an athlete and coach, I have been exposed to some of the top minds in fitness and personal achievement. My clients often ask me what books I read and what resources have proved to be the most valuable to me. I'd like to share that information with you.

One of my first introductions to viewing fat in a whole new light was Covert Bailey's *Fit or Fat* (Boston: Houghton Mifflin, 1978).

The definitive works on the relationship between blood type and food choice are Peter D'Adamo's *Eat Right 4 Your Type* (New York: G. P. Putnam and Sons, 1996) and *Cook Right 4 Your Type* (New York: G. P. Putnam and Sons, 1998).

Richard and Rachael Heller's book, *The Carbohydrate Addict's Diet* (New York: Signet Books, 1991) outlines the dangers of a high-carbohydrate approach to nutrition.

Philip Maffetone's *In Fitness and in Health* (David Barmore Productions, 1997) remains one of the classic "must reads" for the athlete or aspiring athlete interested in getting healthy and fit.

His latest work is *The Maffetone Method* (New York: McGraw-Hill, 1999).

Anyone interested in personal transformation and life-changing insights must immerse himself or herself in the ideas contained in Anthony Robbins's *Awaken the Giant Within: How to Take Immediate Control of Your Mental, Emotional, Physical and Financial Destiny* (New York: Fireside, 1993) and *Unlimited Power: The New Science of Personal Achievement* (New York: Fireside, 1986).

David Seaman's reference book *Clinical Nutrition* (NutrAnalysis, Inc., 1998) is not light reading. It's an amazingly thorough analysis on the role nutrition plays in health and muscular function.

Barry Sears's *The Zone* (New York: ReganBooks, 1995), definitively explains how certain combinations of food influence the role insulin plays in fat storage and undermining health.

Dr. Robert O. Young's *Sick and Tired? Reclaim Your Inner Terrain* (Lindon, Utah: Woodland Publishing, 1999), details the "new biology" that identifies overacidification of the blood as the primary cause of most degenerative diseases.

Applied Kinesiologist Referral Center

The International College of Applied Kinesiology (ICAK), founded by George Goodheart, provides a referral service for anyone interested in locating an ICAK-certified applied kinesiologist. All you need to do is contact the ICAK directly at 913–384–5336, and the organization will provide you with a list of AK specialists in your area.

Products and Services to Alkalize and Energize

The research microbiologist Dr. Robert O. Young of InnerLight Biological Research Center created the Alkalizer

Pack, which includes the Super Greens drink to prevent the overacidification of the blood and surrounding tissues. The drink is a blend of organic concentrated green vegetables, grasses, and grains and comes in either a powder that you mix with water or in capsules. Sipping on this drink throughout the day helps to gently pull the blood and tissue balance from an acid base into a healthy alkaline state.

The drink's ingredients include kamut grass, barleygrass, lemongrass, shavegrass, wheatgrass, alfalfa leaf, dandelion leaf, bilberry leaf, black walnut leaf, blackberry leaf, plaintain leaf, red raspberry leaf, blueberry leaf, boldo leaf, goldenseal leaf, papaya leaf, strawberry leaf, lecithin, white willow leaf, slippery elm bark, marshmallow root, paude arco, cornsilk, rosemary, betatene, rose hip, echinacea purp tops, doggrass, meadowsweet, aloe whole leaf concentrate, oat grass, soy sprout concentrate, kale, spinach, okra, cabbage, celery, parsley leaf, broccoli, watercress, alfalfa-juice concentrate, turmeric, tomato, peppermint leaf, spearmint leaf, wintergreen leaf, sage, thyme, rosemary leaf, and high-frequency mineral complexes.

For specific details on this product, or to order, see the contact information located at the end of the appendix.

Self-Discovery Through Blood Analysis

To me, one of the most exciting new investigative tools in the field of health and fitness is the use of high-powered microscopes to assess the health and function of the blood. The process, called live blood cell analysis and the mycotoxic/oxidative stress test, is performed by a certified microscopist who examines the blood and visually records the change in form and function of the red blood cells, white blood cells, and platelets. He or she draws a few drops of blood from a simple pinprick, places them on a glass slide, and views them under a microscope. The images are projected onto a television monitor for you and the microscopist to observe and discuss. If you're in optimal health, you will see how round and clear a healthy red blood cell looks, how active and purposeful the white blood cells act, and how clear the plasma appears. Under stressful conditions, including emotional or physical stress and poor dietary practices, such as the consumption of too much sugar, caffeine, alcohol, or protein, the blood turns acidic, promoting the growth of bacteria, yeast, mold, and fungal forms, which can be seen during these fascinating glimpses into the blood. In the mycotoxic/oxidative stress test, the microscopist can detect specific areas of organization and disorganization, such an imbalance in the reproductive organs, by examining one drop of dry blood.

For more information about the Alkalizer Pack, which includes the Super Greens drink, or live blood cell analysis and the mycotoxic/oxidative stress test, contact my office at 800–913–9266, e-mail info@worldultrafit.com or visit my Website at www.worldultrafit.com